AWAKENING *with* SANSKRIT

Introduction to
THE *SACRED LANGUAGE* OF YOGA

KATY POOLE, PH.D.

Cover design: *JVP Consulting*

Book & eBook design and layout: *JVP Consulting, Big Fish Marketing*

Original Sanskrit translations: *Katy "Katyayani" Poole, Ph.D.*

Special thanks to: *Christine Komenda, layout assistance and emotional support*

ISBN-13: 978-1463731144

First Edition Printing: *February 2007*

Second Edition Printing: *April 2009*

Third Edition Printing: *July 2011*

Printed in the USA

Sanskrit for Yoga

A Note on Sanskrit Transliteration

For the ease of comprehension for beginning students of Sanskrit, I have deliberately not employed the conventional academic transliteration of Sanskrit words to avoid confusing English readers. Instead, I've adopted a more colloquial rendering of such terms.

A Disclaimer

The information presented in this volume is meant to make general comparisons of Sanskrit (as it is understood in the Vedic traditions) with linguistic and scientific theories. I acknowledge the complexities within contemporary linguistics and physics and that they are systems of knowledge under constant revision, refinement and discovery. My remarks, therefore, could be mistakenly regarded as overly simplistic, naive or open to debate. However, my intention here is to simply open a conversation that widens the relevance of Sanskrit beyond the narrow confines of elite academia and to inspire yoga practitioners to receive it on a sacred and practical level.

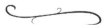

Also by Dr. Katy Poole

- *Feeling the Shakti of Sanskrit™*

- *Sanskrit for Yogis™: Introduction to Nada*

- *The Alphabet of the Body™*

- *Sanskrit & Yoga Mastery Program™*

For additional information send email or visit online locations:

- *Sanskrit For Yoga LLC:*

    - *info@SanskritForYoga.com*

    - *www.SanskritForYoga.com*

    - *www.SanskritCourses.com*

- *Dr Katy Poole LLC:*

    - *info@DrKatyPoole.com*

    - *www.DrKatyPoole.com*

    - *www.VedicAstrologyLifeInsight.com*

Testimonials

"At last! A Yogic approach to learning Sanskrit, the language at the basis of our practice...it will reveal the sheer beauty of the Sanskrit Language and its deep expression of the spiritual." ~ **Judith Hanson Lasater, Ph.D., PT, Yoga Teacher (since 1971), Author of** *A Year of Living Your Yoga*

"This profound approach to Sanskrit is of great value to anyone who wants to experience more deeply the power of mantra, chant, and to investigate for themselves the sacred science encoded in the language of yoga." ~ **Sally Kempton, Meditation Teacher,** *Swami Durgananda,* **Author of** *Meditation for the Love of It*

"I so appreciate how you present Sanskrit in a sacred manner that gives a novice confidence and inspiration to begin the path. This is a jewel in the lotus of educational material recommended to all." ~ **Shiva Rea, M.A., Yoga Teacher, Sacred Activist**

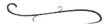

Dedication

For all the great seers, the rishis, whose extraordinary realization enhanced the world with the art and science of the Vedas in Sanskrit. And for all my teachers, their teachers, and all who taught before them who kept the knowledge of the seers unbroken for centuries so that all yogis can partake in its splendor.

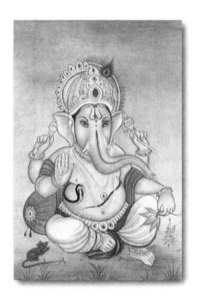

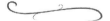

Contents

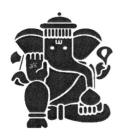

Introduction

My Discovery of Sanskrit, the Technology of Awakening Higher States of Consciousness

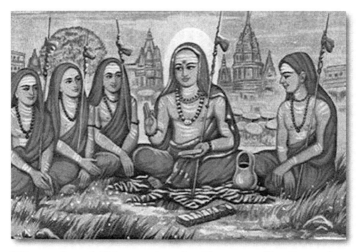

"Every day children sat under the spreading branches of an ancient banyan tree and recited the Vedic texts after their teacher." ~ from the *Kena Upanishad*

My mouth hung agape. It seemed impossible for someone to lift off the ground and defy gravity. I couldn't imagine not eating for a single day, let alone years. I always wanted to make myself invisible, but never knew how. By the time I finished the final chapter of Paramahansa Yogananda's *Autobiography of Yogi*, I made a firm decision: *I wanted to become enlightened.*

Yogananda's stories of yogis and saints who'd attained heightened states of consciousness and miraculous abilities through yoga and meditation filled me with wonder. As I surveyed the mundane possibilities of my life, I found nothing more worthwhile than the pursuit of liberation from all physical and mental limitations. I questioned everything and the answer – a haunting whisper -- always came back the same: *There's something more incredible in this life that beckons you.*

Just 18-years-old, I was fiery, idealistic, and spunky. College mostly bored me, except for my South Indian music and African dance classes, which stirred a vibrant longing within me. I needed a Guru. I made my next decision.

I'd drop out of college, travel to the Himalayas and find an enlightened sage who'd help me realize my limitless power within. It sounded reasonable enough to me when I explained this plan to my family. My mother, however, was mortified.

"Just where do you think you're going, young lady, to find this so-called goo-roo?" My quest, it seemed, was not as obviously important to everyone as it was to me.

"Kathmandu, Nepal," I quipped as if every teenager in America was going there as the new hip hangout. It was 1988 and globalization was still in its infancy. Nepal may as well have been the moon.

Although many objections were raised, I refused to listen to any argument that presented an obstacle. Nothing could hold me back from what I wanted most in the world. I was convinced that Nepal, at the base of the holy Himalayan mountains, was the place I'd find it. As I boarded the plane to Kathmandu, I promised myself: *I won't return to the United States until I've achieved enlightenment!*

Arriving in Nepal, the plane circled the city as barefoot peasants shooed some errant cows off the runway and finally came in to land. Out of the airport gates, I stepped toward my destiny. I also happened to step in a pile of dung, slipping and falling to the ground. A crowd gathered and laughed unashamedly at my predicament.

Now I understand why. Here was a silly young girl, wielding an oversized backpack, so intent on getting somewhere that she couldn't be bothered to look where she stepped. A kind-looking gentleman offered me his hand.

"Welcome to Nepal," he said brightly. "Why are you here?"

When I told him my plan, he displayed the same incredulous look my family had worn. "What is there in enlightenment?" he questioned. "You're an American. You have everything. There is nothing for you in Nepal!"

Then handing me a card, he concluded, "Call these people. They can help you."

As soon as I arrived at my guesthouse, I read the card's inscription: *United States Peace Corps: Nepali Language Immersions.* The helpful stranger gave me a tip that I hadn't even considered. If I were to meet an enlightened yogi, speaking the native language could prove indispensable. I promptly enrolled.

Following a week of Nepali classes and a barrage of personal questions, my teacher, Shankar Narayan, ordered me to gather my things. It was very unusual – and quite improper -- for Nepalis to see a young woman traveling by herself and staying alone. I learned this the day before when I shared that I was interned at the *Hotel Shiva,* a reputed dump of a place housing a coterie of ex-patriots who'd left America during the Nixon administration. Shankar turned pale at my confession and gasped, "Oh, no! That's not a place for a lady to stay."

Immediately following my tutorial, Shankar Narayan hailed a taxi, hauled my bags down the stairs of the *Hotel Shiva,* and gestured for me to get in the back. I had no idea where he was taking me.

We bumped along the narrow streets of Kathmandu, dodging stray cattle, erratic bicyclists, and kids playing crude games of cricket. Then the road opened out of the city toward the village Balaju. I drank in the beauty of purple morning glories set against emerald rice paddies. My eyes met the sweet glance of water buffaloes as they waded up to their floppy ears in irrigation canals. I admired the grace of women working in the paddies, swaying in their red saris like a dance. And I swooned at the scent of incense wafting from a small roadside shrine next to an ancient tree.

I thought I'd entered some form of paradise that the rest of the world had lost in its pursuit of "progress." I remembered the small suburban town in which I'd grown up, in contrast, where no one was ever home, where lawns were mowed with gas machines, and where the only form of animal life was securely fastened to a leash and taken out to politely relieve itself twice a day on the carefully manicured grass. For the first time in my life, I felt I'd arrived home thousands of miles from where I'd grown up.

No sooner had that feeling entered my heart, than the taxi stopped at a three-storied cement building. As we approached the entrance, a newborn calf ran out the front door toward its mother in the courtyard. Shankar Narayan nodded to me remarking, "An auspicious sign for you." A man resembling an older, grayer version of Shankar, welcomed us with palms together: *Namaste*.

"Uncle, I've brought an American student to live with you," Shankar announced plaintively.

"Good, good," was all the man said. "Please come."

Over a tin cup of steaming milk tea, I learned that Shankar Narayan's uncle was the head priest of the most important Hindu temple in Kathmandu. Whole-heartedly invited to stay as long as I wanted, I was instantly treated like a long-lost daughter. Never in my life had I experienced so much love given by complete strangers to a complete stranger. The Nepali hospitality heaped on me by Krishna Narayan and his family changed me forever.

Offered a room to myself on the first floor of the home, a place of honor next to the family shrine room, every morning at 4:00 a.m. a loud cacophony of strange and rhythmic sounds awakened me. These beautiful, hypnotic, and nonsensical melodies put my mind at rest. My breathing became deep and full. I relaxed totally into the pleasant pulse of warm electricity coursing through my body. Letting go, I forgot the time. Not quite asleep and not quite awake, I entered a natural state of meditation.

My biorhythms quickly adjusted to this morning routine. I found it easy to awake much earlier than I was accustomed, eager to experience the "music" again and again. As soon as Krishna Uncle and his little boy, Babu, had settled in the shrine room, I'd sneak over to the side of the doorway and seat myself in full lotus posture. As their voices grew stronger, faster, and yet precisely rhythmic, I'd dissolve into the sweet sensations that led me to a vast open space within. It felt pure there. I experienced a wakeful awareness that contained no thought. The best way I found to express it was through a blissful smile spread across my face.

"You like our *adhyayanam*?" Krishna Uncle asked me one morning.

Is that what this is called? I wondered to myself. *Adhyaa-yaa-num*?

"I don't know," I answered. "I've never heard this before."

"It is teacher-disciple method," he explained. "I sit. You sit. I chant. You listen. You repeat."

And that's what I did for many, many mornings before I ever learned that I was chanting in Sanskrit. All I knew was that these pure impulses of sound were what energized, enlivened, and awakened my yoga and meditation practice. After chanting, I became so acutely aware of the structures of my subtle body (*marmas, nadis, and cakras*) that pulsed with renewed *prana* (subtle life-force). Spontaneously, my body formed the shapes of the yoga *asanas*. And my mind and emotions became silent and still.

Once Krishna Uncle was in a very revealing mood. We were sitting together on the roof of his house on low jute stools. It was kite-flying season in Kathmandu and the sky was full of flourish. For many months, I had asked him about enlightenment to no avail. He'd never answer a single one of my questions. He'd just shake his head slightly side to side with his eyes cast up, as if I'd asked something very good, as if the question alone was sufficient. But that day on the roof, Krishna Uncle felt like talking.

"You know Sanskrit is not a language," he explained. "It is the very mind of God. This world is the spoken breath of God. Our breath is the breath of God. When we direct it back to the divine source with our holy chants, we merge with Him."

I nodded in agreement. Krishna Uncle's words perfectly described what I experienced as I first heard and felt the sounds of Sanskrit. "Is Sanskrit the secret behind enlightenment?" I queried sincerely.

"Yes, correct." Krishna Uncle responded. "You become very intelligent by intoning these sounds. Your mind becomes very clear and open. Your heart becomes happy. The family relations improve. And your life's duty is easily fulfilled."

I knew I'd discovered the secret behind yoga's power to achieve higher states of consciousness and enlightenment. I decided then and there I would dedicate myself to perfecting the art of Vedic chanting in Sanskrit to open myself more to this sweet experience of awakening.

Then one day, Krishna Uncle approached me with a look of concern. "You are not educated," he remarked. "Who will respect you?"

I became confused. *Respect? Why did that matter to me?*

Yet Krishna Uncle persisted in his worry. Finally, he spoke directly. "You must finish your education. It is essential."

"But the only thing I want to learn is what I'm learning here," I argued.

"You can earn your degree in Sanskrit studies," he reasoned. "Then you will be found credible."

After several weeks going back and forth like this, I finally conceded. I'd return to the United States to pursue my studies in Sanskrit. Keeping my word, I enrolled in the Sanskrit program offered through the Department of Religious Studies at the University of California, Santa Barbara.

Initially there were 25 students in my academic Sanskrit class, which even on the first day was brutally difficult. It reminded me of the day my father taught me to ski – *by pushing me down the hill!* Nothing about the way Sanskrit was taught in the university remotely resembled my shrine room lessons at Krishna Uncle's home. I felt like I accidently walked in on a theoretical physics class that demanded rigorous understanding of calculus as a pre-requisite. I checked my schedule. No, this was the right room. And this was Sanskrit class.

On the second day of class, only five students showed up. By the third day, attendance had dwindled to just three of us. The only reason I remained was because my teacher, Mrs. Nandini Iyer, pulled me aside whispering, "Only those with good past-life merit are able to learn Sanskrit." She stoked my fire. I certainly was going to be one of those with good past-life merit!

The grammatical structure of Sanskrit is so intricate, complex and difficult, it's a miracle that I had the dedication and discipline to stick it out for five years. In fact, I performed well enough in my studies to be accepted into the masters and doctorate program in the Department of Religious Studies at the University of California, Santa Barbara.

Yet I longed to experience Sanskrit as it had been orally transmitted from teacher to student for thousands of years. Although I had gained proficiency in grammar and translation, I felt that the sacred status and enlightening power of Sanskrit had been totally lost with the academic, "dead classical language" approach. I wanted to immerse myself in the oral transmission of the sacred language from teacher to student as I had in Nepal and re-enliven it in my spiritual practice.

At that point, I had studied hard, labored in my understanding of grammar and syntax, and memorized multitudes of complex rules, paradigms, and declensions. I was quite confident I was going to become a great Sanskrit and yoga master! Fortunately, I received a grant to return to India for five years to study with traditional Sanskrit teachers. Receiving the grant was relatively easy. Finding a teacher who'd accept a non-Brahmin, unmarried, American woman as a student was another matter.

I sent out over a hundred letters to potential teachers and not one was answered. I understood that it was uncustomary for a Brahmin male master of Sanskrit to impart the sacred transmission of Vedic chanting to an American woman. Krishna Uncle had made a great exception by teaching me, which I hadn't fully appreciated at the time. For all other traditional teachers, it appeared, I simply did not fulfill the purity and caste requirements that forbid anyone but a Brahmin male to chant the auspicious Vedas in Sanskrit.

I almost gave up in despair when a letter arrived from India. It was addressed to me by a Sanskrit *pandita* (scholar), Abhijit Chattopadyay, who informed me that he wasn't interested at first in accepting me as a student. But then he had two dreams that convinced him otherwise. In the first dream, his teacher appeared to him telling him that if this knowledge had been kept in the hands of women it would never be lost! And in the second dream, he envisioned a foreign woman teaching many women students of yoga Vedic chanting in Sanskrit. In his letter, he described them as "oceans of ladies." So I'd passed the first test and found a suitable teacher.

The traditional way of studying Sanskrit required that I live with my teacher and become part of his family as I had in Nepal with Krishna Uncle's family. And that's what I did. When I arrived in the city of Calcutta, I hired a cycle rickshaw to take me to the home of my teacher. It was some time after my arrival that Panditji gave me my first lesson. Initially, I was expected to help clean his modest home, take care of guests, sweep the courtyard, and run errands. I was naturally frustrated, thinking that perhaps I was invited to be a servant and not a student like I'd expected. I was still very arrogant about my academic accomplishments and my intelligence.

Finally after several weeks, Panditji asked if I'd recite a simple line in Sanskrit. I thought, *"This is so easy. I'm really going to make great progress. I can translate this. I can tell all the different parts of speech and analyze the grammar."* With confidence, I pronounced the first word.

The sound had barely escaped my lips when my teacher blocked his ears and said, "Oh, this is terrible! It's the worst Sanskrit I've ever heard in my life! You must start at the beginning."

I thought, *"What does he mean? How can he not be impressed with me? I've spent so much time studying Sanskrit. Surely, I'm no beginner!"*

But beginner I became. For more than six months I was only permitted to chant the 50 syllables of the Sanskrit alphabet every day and nothing more advanced. I thought I'd go insane. The repetition for eight hours or more per day was maddening. Just when I thought I'd perfected a sound, Panditji would clap his hands and make me repeat it again and again, each time discovering a new flaw.

In India, it's traditional that teachers don't tell you the reason you're given certain tasks. If you ask why, you'll be told, "Yes, you will chant." And then if you ask again, "But why do I have to chant the same sounds over and over again, every day for months and months?" My teacher always answered simply, "You will chant it. No problem."

I was so discouraged, humiliated, and full of despair. According to tradition, you can't just dump your teacher because you don't like his or her method. You have to persevere. You have to give up your ego in order to make any kind of progress in yoga and meditation. As a student you must realize that you're not in charge.

Indians naturally understand the guru-disciple relationship. Recently when I was in India, I stood outside a temple where I met an accomplished yogi. He asked me why I'd come to India and I explained that I'd brought a group of yoga teachers to experience her sacred culture on the Chardham Pilgrimage. He responded mockingly, "No one in America is a yoga teacher, much less a yogi!"

I asked him to explain why he felt that way, though I already knew the answer from my own experience. He shared, "When I was learning from my Guru he only permitted me to perform one yoga *asana* and that was *tadasana*! I practiced it every day for 12 years."

Then he showed me his perfected posture. It amazed me. His body became a column of pure light and radiance. His mastery of yoga was not a physical attainment, but achieved through the abandonment of ego, self-identification and pride.

Following the path of many yogis before me who faced equally humiliating and ego-defying exercises imposed upon them by their teachers, I gave up struggling against what I thought was a ridiculous waste of my time. I surrendered. Surrender to the teacher is the most important part of learning anything sacred. You have to let go of your ego and accept the authority of one who knows more than you. As an American, this was extremely hard for me.

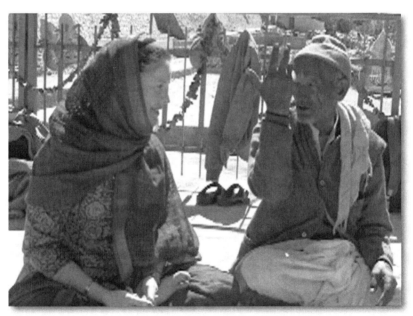

Dr. Poole with Vedic Pandit at the Source of the Ganges (Gangotri, India)

INTRODUCTION TO THE SACRED LANGUAGE OF YOGA

When I finally allowed myself to accept the method of learning imposed on me, I placed all my attention on mindfully experiencing the pure sounds of Sanskrit. I observed that they had a sublimely pleasant effect on my nervous system. I discovered a deep bliss vibrating from the core of my being. And I came to love that simple practice of chanting the primordial sounds of Sanskrit without worrying about what they meant or how much progress I was making.

Eventually, I realized the method behind my teacher's madness. By the continuous daily chanting of Sanskrit, I determined its supreme value in attaining the goal of yoga. It opens the channels of higher perception, increases the flow of *prana*, cultivates deep awareness and functioning of the subtle nervous system, and awakens the state of enlightened consciousness.

At the end of six months, my teacher finally said, "Now your voice has *shakti* in it. Now your voice has energy and power in it. Now I can teach you."

That moment became a revelation for me. I knew then that Sanskrit is not an old, dead, classical language that only accomplished academics can decipher. Instead, it became for me a living technology for awakening higher states of consciousness, understanding the subtle laws of creation, and attaining advanced states of meditation leading to enlightenment.

I spent five years in India receiving the traditional transmission of Sanskrit as sacred sound and meeting many saints and masters of yoga. In my meetings and studies, I discovered that Sanskrit (at the basis of the formal practices of yoga) transmutes the body and mind from the identification with the ego as the separate I-sense to the dawning of a presence that fills the Being with transcendental light.

Twelve years after meeting Krishna Narayan in Nepal and hearing Sanskrit for the first time, I earned a masters degree in Sanskrit and a doctorate in Religious Studies and devised a method of teaching Sanskrit, which I coined *Sanskrit for Yogis*™.

The *Sanskrit for Yogis*™ method relies on the simple and profound tradition of imparting the language of enlightenment orally from teacher-to-student instruction as I learned from my teachers in Nepal and India. Its purpose is to cultivate a refined opening of the subtle physiology, leading to the awakening of higher states of awareness, the goal of yoga and meditation.

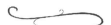

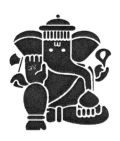

Chapter One
Sanskrit: The Language of Yoga and Enlightenment

"If the sun has set, the moon has set, and the fire has gone out, by what light does a person see?" King Janaka asked his Guru, Yajnavalkya.

He answered, "If the sun has set, the moon has set, and the fire has gone out, a person sees by the light of the Self."
~ from the Brihadaranyaka Upanishad

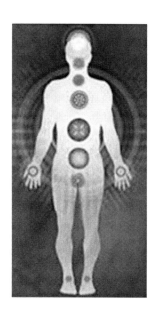

There's something amazing about the Sanskrit language: *It's the foundation of all Indo-European languages.* That means if you speak English, French, German, Russian or any European language (with the exception of Hungarian) as well as many of the modern Indian languages and Persian, Sanskrit is at the root.

At some point in history there may have been a common language, Sanskrit, spoken by a vast population of people spread out over a diverse geography. As a result, many, many of our words in English derive from Sanskrit roots. If when you come across Sanskrit words in yoga, you can make that connection, the meaning of the seemingly foreign words becomes familiar.

For example, "Sanskrit" is the anglicized form of the word for the sacred language of yoga, *samskrta*, consisting of two parts: *sam* and *krta*.

Sam sounds like our English word "sum," and has the same meaning of "total."

Krta has the same meaning as our English word, "created."

Together, the word *samskrta* means "created" or "made" out of the state of the "total," or "unity."

Samskrta is not just a word that has a symbolic meaning. *It's an expression of the structure of the material world that's echoed in modern science.* Quantum physics, for example, reveals in String Theory that everything in the objective, material universe is vibrating at its core. What seems solid and unchanging in our physical world is actually moving so quickly that it appears to be standing still. This implies that if you were subtle enough in your awareness, you'd be able to "hear" and "see" those vibrations and replicate them with your voice.

The theory that distinguishable and varied vibrations form the core of all created matter lies at the basis of the Sanskrit language. Most importantly, Sanskrit is a technology that achieves something remarkable: *By replicating the subtle sounds of creation with the human voice, one becomes unified with all aspects of the physical and subtle universe.*

The ancient sages of India (known as *rishis* or "seers of ultimate truth") made this discovery of Sanskrit by attaining extraordinary states of intelligent perception through meditation. Their expanded consciousness permitted them to see and hear the subtle "strings of code" at the basis of creation. They recorded these arrangements of sounds in their speech, committed them to memory, and passed them down to their disciples to preserve them for posterity. The sounds they heard were combinations of the 50 Sanskrit syllables, forming the corpus of the Veda.

The word "Veda" comes from the same Sanskrit verbal root from which we get our English word, "video." Just like a video is a projection of pixilations of light and sound, this world is a diversified array of vibrations, distinguishing themselves only by different combinations of sounds and rhythms.

The *rishis* saw in their mind's eye that these subtle sounds abide at the very source of all things manifest in nature -- like trees, rocks, plants, animals and human beings. They then recorded what they saw and heard in the form of rhythmic speech, or *mantras*, which make up what are sometimes called the "hymns" of the Veda. You could say that the chants of the Veda are recordings of the way the created world arises, mutates, and dissolves.

These *mantras*, or pure forms of sound, are likened to sonic building blocks that construct the underlying architecture of both the visible and subtle realms. When you replicate these *mantras* exactly as they have been passed down orally in the Vedic tradition, they cultivate your subtle nervous system to that of the extraordinarily intelligent and perceptive *rishis*. You gain the same ability to perceive nature at its source.

The oral transmission of nature's vibrational code has been kept alive for thousands of generations in India through the sacred Guru-disciple relationship[*]. The teacher enlivens the liberating energy in the student's body-mind through the constant repetition of Sanskrit. Beginning when a child is just four or five-years-old, she memorizes thousands of rhythmic patterns by mimicking her teacher's tone, pattern of breath, and pronunciation. This continues daily for twelve years, during which time the child's nervous system is cultured to perceive more subtle levels of reality – from the physical to the vital inner core of all things. Purified by the continuous pulse of healing sound, her body itself effortlessly channels a higher light. And through the breath's regulation by proper pronunciation of the Sanskrit syllables, her mind is directed to a more clairvoyant and clairaudient perception of conscious thought.

---

[*] I've also attempted to maintain it authentically in my *Sanskrit for Yogis Method*™.

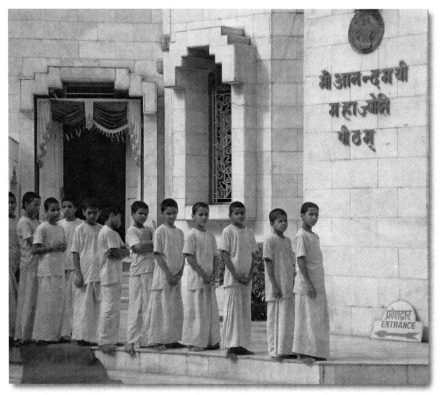

Young Sanskrit Students at the Samadhi Shrine of Anandamayi Ma (Haridwar, India)

When the child-disciple reaches physical maturity by the age of 16 or so, her very body has become a beacon of healing, vitalizing, and bliss-bestowing light by this ancient method of Sanskrit chanting. Such an enlightened individual is invaluable to everything within her vicinity. She instills an environment of peace by her very presence, fostering the growth of positive human values in the society at large. The plants and animals likewise respond in harmony with such a state of being.

For this reason, the *Hatha Yoga Pradipika* asserts that "the union of the mind with pure sound is the highest and most subtle form of yoga." Chanting Sanskrit is an essential and complementary practice to yoga *asana*, *pranayama*, and meditation, the benefit of which is for a much larger field of influence beyond the physical body and mind.

I never fully appreciated the value of chanting Sanskrit and practicing yoga and meditation for anyone other than myself. Like most westerners, I wanted enlightenment for personal gains. I wanted a yogic body to look good. I wanted peace of mind so I could negotiate my relationships with minimal emotional annoyance. And I persisted in my Sanskrit studies because it made meditation an effortless practice for me. I enjoyed the bliss.

It wasn't until I spent several months living in a small central Indian village along the Narmada River with, Nani, Babita Verma's grandmother, that my mind expanded. Village homes are crowded scenes. I had no personal space, even sleeping in a bed with five other women. I understood why yogis ran away to meditate in the remote Himalayas. You simply can't find a place to practice without being disturbed in traditional India!

I discovered an abandoned storeroom, however, in Nani's house that became my practice space. I thought I would escape notice there and conduct my daily practices without interruption. This lasted only a day before my secret was out. The following morning, as I swooped my arms above my head in the first *vinyasa* of my sun salutation, I noticed a crowd had gathered outside the room. Many sets of eyes were peeping through the window. Ignoring them, I continued with my yoga, chanting, and meditation practice. I thought they'd get the "hint" and leave me to myself for a while.

Yet once my practice was over and I left the room for breakfast, the crowd persisted, stopping me with a multitude of varied requests.

"My son is getting married. Will you look at the photos of potential brides for him?"

"My mother-in-law is very sick. Could you pronounce a healing *mantra* for her?"

"*Didi* (sister), will you bless our seeds? We want to have a good crop this year. Last year was terrible."

I found this a truly strange spectacle. I had no idea why these villagers felt that I could help with their problems, when Nani made it clear. "You are a *yogini* who's come to the village. Your presence here is a blessing for the people and the land. Such a *yogini* purifies the place by her meditation and her chanting of Vedas. She brings God here."

My attitude changed from then on. The practice of yoga, meditation, and chanting Sanskrit *mantras* took on an entirely different meaning for me. It inspires, uplifts and enlivens nature and its inhabitants, establishing a positive and healthy environment for everyone within the vicinity of the practicing yogi. I've come to appreciate these practices not only for my own peace of mind, but also for peace on Earth.

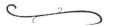

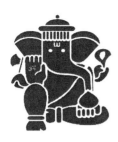

Chapter Two
Name and Form in Sanskrit and in the Practice of Yoga Asana

The divine name is the pure nectar of bliss.
~ Swami Muktananda

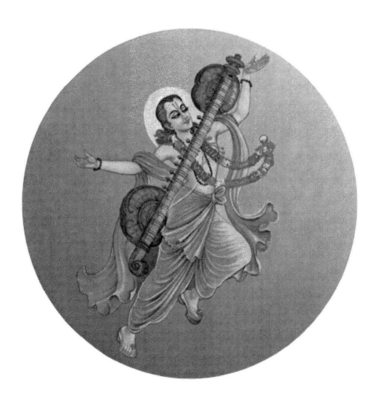

Many times students will ask me what a word in Sanskrit means in English. I myself spent many years pouring over a thick dictionary in vain attempts at rendering the intricate, poetic beauty of Sanskrit into plain, direct and comprehensible English. Yet how can you describe what chocolate tastes like if you've never tasted chocolate?

Throughout my traditional studies with teachers in India, I had ample opportunities to distinguish the noticeable and unique feelings of each of the 50 syllables in Sanskrit and their combinations. I'd feel specific channels of energy in my subtle body open when I'd pronounce a letter or a *mantra* perfectly. I wondered if the current of energy contained within every word in Sanskrit and its directional pattern had some relationship to the shape of what it represented in nature.

Through self-study, I observed when I'd say the Sanskrit name for a yoga posture, I'd detect a flow of energy along a circuit of channels in my body. When I'd make the shape of the posture physically, its alignment matched the flow of the syllable's subtle energetic current.

In Sanskrit, the name and form of anything are identical. This is not the case with modern languages. The words we express in English don't participate in the vibrational structure of those things. Instead, they are symbolic.

For example, if I were to gather a group of English speakers and ask them to tell me the first word that arises in their mind when I say "apple," they'd offer so many different responses. Some will think, "red." Others will think, "crunchy." Still others will think, "tree, juicy, computer, and so on."

Everyone would conjure a different association of just one word in English. I'd be obliged to explain what I mean by "apple." I'd have to use many more words to create a symbolic vision in everyone's mind until we could all arrive at a common understanding. Even then, there'd be the possibility for different symbolic associations. Imagine in one conversation how much misunderstanding there is! It's no wonder we don't have peace on earth. There is so much division in our language.

In Sanskrit, this is not the case. Instead, the name of something is always identical with the form.

There are probably a hundred different words for "apple" in Sanskrit. If I were to say "apple" in Sanskrit, the word I'd invoke would match the vibrational structure of the kind of apple I had in mind. In other words, the syllables would replicate the sounds that constitute the subtle, energetic form of the object being spoken. Everyone would understand immediately what I was talking about. Our minds would unify around the vibrations of the word/object.

Because name and form are identical in Sanskrit, pronouncing the Sanskrit names for the yoga postures becomes vitally important to your progress in the practice of yoga. This is because the name embodies the energetic shape that is replicated in the gross physical body, which is at its source a vibrating mass of sound pulsations.

Specifically, these sound pulsations are localized along 107 points on our physical body called *marmas*. If you've ever had an acupuncture treatment, you'll understand what a *marma* is. An acupuncturist determines where the energetic block is located in the internal structure of the body that is causing the symptom. She then inserts a needle into one or more points on the body's surface that connects with the area of stagnancy through subtle channels. The pressure on those points sends an energetic flow from the surface to the inner and subtle structures of the body, enlivening a connection that promotes health and wholeness.

In Chinese medicine, these energetic gateways that open to the deep recesses of the body are called "meridian points," which derive from the *marma* points put forth by the older Indian medical system of Ayurveda. Ayurveda maps a set of 107[*] sensitive *marma* points on the body's surface that connect via subtle channels (*nadis*) to the deeper energetic centers of the nervous system known as *cakras*. Each *marma* point has a Sanskrit syllable associated with it. When a Sanskrit syllable is pronounced perfectly it sends an energetic current through its *marma* point, enlivening a pathway to invigorate the core of the central nervous system.

When you say the name for a yoga posture in Sanskrit, you emit a pulse of *prana* or life force along a series of *marma* points associated with those sounds. The physical alignment of a posture, therefore, has a "sonic shape" that correlates with it and replicates the energetic core of the thing in nature your body is forming.

The ancient yogis observed nature very closely. They noted the pattern of breath in creatures and plants when their bodies formed certain shapes. The yogis replicated those patterns with their own bodies, matching their breath to the breath of the creature they imitated. The Sanskrit name for that posture perfectly matches the "shape" of the creature's life force as it corresponds to the relevant *marma* points and associated Sanskrit syllables on the human body. Pronouncing the Sanskrit name for the posture and feeling its energetic flow,

---

[*] There is a debate in Ayurveda which also places the number at 117.

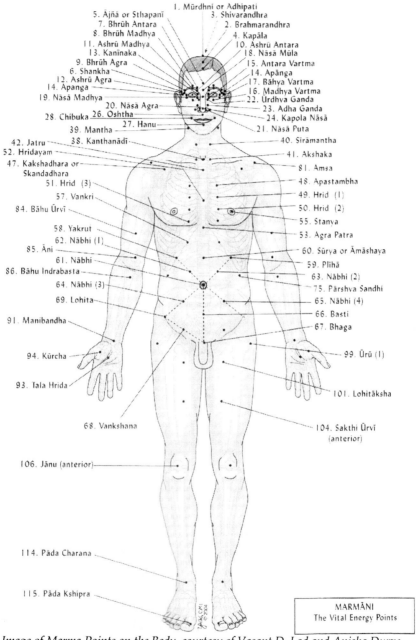

1. Mūrdhni or Adhipati
5. Ājñā or Sthapanī
3. Shivarandhra
7. Bhrüh Antara
2. Brahmarandhra
8. Bhrüh Madhya
4. Kapāla
11. Ashrü Madhya
10. Ashrü Antara
13. Kanīnaka
18. Nāsā Müla
9. Bhrüh Agra
15. Antara Vartma
6. Shankha
14. Apānga
12. Ashrü Agra
17. Bāhya Vartma
14. Apanga
16. Madhya Vartma
19. Nāsā Madhya
22. Urdhva Ganda
20. Nāsā Agra
23. Adha Ganda
28. Chibuka 26. Oshtha
24. Kapola Nāsā
27. Hanu
39. Mantha
21. Nāsā Puta
42. Jatru 38. Kanthanādī
40. Sīrāmantha
52. Hridayam
41. Akshaka
47. Kakshadhara or
81. Amsa
    Skandadhara
48. Apastambha
51. Hrid (3)
49. Hrid (1)
57. Vankri
50. Hrid (2)
84. Bāhu Ūrvī
55. Stanya
58. Yakrut
53. Agra Patra
62. Nābhi (1)
85. Āni
60. Sūrya or Āmāshaya
61. Nābhi
59. Plīhā
86. Bāhu Indrabasta
63. Nābhi (2)
64. Nābhi (3)
75. Pārshva Sandhi
69. Lohita
65. Nābhi (4)
66. Basti
91. Manibandha
67. Bhaga
94. Kürcha
99. Ūrū (1)
93. Tala Hrida
101. Lohitāksha
68. Vankshana
104. Sakthi Ūrvī
    (anterior)
106. Jānu (anterior)
114. Pāda Charana
115. Pāda Kshipra

MARMĀNI
The Vital Energy Points

Image of Marma Points on the Body courtesy of Vasant D. Lad and Anisha Durve,
Marma Points of Ayurveda (Albuquerque, 2008).

therefore, is the power behind your yoga practice to achieve its ultimate goal: *absolute unity with everything in nature.*

For example, the name for "cobra pose" in Sanskrit is *bhujanga* consisting of the syllables *bham, um, jam, gam, nam* and *am. Bhujanga* is the physical and sonic form of a specific type of cobra with its body coiled and its hood extended. The syllables that make up the name for such a creature are identical to its form. The *asana* shape replicates the physical form of such a snake, whereas the Sanskrit syllables making up its name replicate its sonic form traced along the *marma* points associated with those syllables.

The *marma* points that correspond with *bham* are located in the center of the chest at the nipples. *Um* are the points right behind the ears. The first syllable of the cobra pose, *bhum,* therefore, traces an energetic flow of *prana* from the center of the chest to the point right behind the ears.

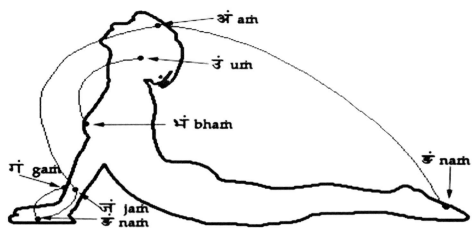

Cobra Posture with Marmas and Corresponding Sanskrit Syllables

The *marma* points in the center of the palms of the hands and feet connect with the *nam* sound. *Gam* and *jam* vibrate in the center of the right and left forearms respectively and *am* is at the top of the head, in the center of the skull.

INTRODUCTION TO THE SACRED LANGUAGE OF YOGA

Envision yourself making the form of a cobra. You'll feel the energy flow from the *marma* points in the center of the chest to the back of the ears. Then lightly press your palms into the earth, extending your feet outward behind the body. You'll then feel the energy rise up through the center of the hands and feet, to the forearms, and to the top of the head.

Every Sanskrit name for the yoga postures creates a similar kind of sonic shape traced along the *marma* points, which match the energetic flow of all forms in nature that you can replicate with your body and breath. And interestingly, the cues that yoga teachers provide to properly align you in the posture follow the sequence of syllables exactly. When learning the yoga postures and how to teach them properly, it is indispensable, therefore, to master the Sanskrit names and their associated *marma* points.

I discovered the connection between the *marma* points, the Sanskrit syllables, and the names for the yoga postures quite by accident. I had often been asked by well-meaning yoga teachers to help them with their Sanskrit pronunciation of the yoga *asanas*. Simply saying the names without the full experience of the energy contained within them seemed unfulfilling to me. There had to be a deeper significance. Pronouncing the names correctly had to serve the goal of yoga: *to establish the body, breath, and mind in unity with all forms in nature.*

I wondered if the ancient treatises on yoga could shed light on the relationship between the Sanskrit names of the yoga postures and the pattern of energy generated by pronouncing them. I first turned to Patanjali's *Yoga Sutras* as they are the most important source of traditional knowledge about yoga. Yet he only devotes three *sutras* to the explanation of *asana*. He states:

Asana should be steady (sthira) and comfortable (sukha). It is achieved by reducing the restless tendency and by identifying with infinity (ananta). Then one remains undisturbed by dualities. ~ **Yoga Sutras 2:46-248** ~

Apart from these three *sutras*, Patanjali doesn't describe the myriad postures that contemporary yogis practice. He provides no instruction toward the attainment of proper *asana*. Instead, Patanjali devotes his treatise to the subject of *samadhi* as the goal of yoga, realized through the repetition of the supreme *mantra, Om*. Sacred sound in Sanskrit clearly takes precedence over physical practices in classical yoga.

The *Hatha Yoga Pradipika* of Svatmarama deals more specifically with the bodily basis of yoga. Hatha Yoga, stemming from the Tantric traditions made popular and public in medieval India, espouses the sacred power contained within the human body and nervous system. The body is a gateway leading to the attainment of enlightened immortality, obtained through mastery of hearing the inner, mystical sounds resonant within the central nervous system. Svatmarama concludes, in fact, "the union of the mind with pure sound is the highest form of yoga." All the cleansing rituals, yoga postures, breathing practices and meditation disciplines described in the *Hatha Yoga Pradipika* simply allow the yogi to listen more deeply to the vibrations abiding at the source of Being and ultimately to merge his awareness with them.

My quest for understanding the relationship between the Sanskrit names for the yoga postures was still not complete. My inquiry led me to the works of the 10th century Kashmir Shaivite mystic, Abhinavagupta, whose massive *Tantraloka* contains profound linkages of the Sanskrit syllables to the structures of the subtle human physiology. I discovered that Abhinavagupta's descriptions of *kundalini*, the *cakra* system, the *nadis*, and *marmas* and their relationship to the energetics of Sanskrit were based in part on *Dhanurveda*, the ancient system of Vedic martial arts.

The *Sushruta Samhita* (c. 4th century), the principle text of *Dhanurveda*, maps 107 vital points on the human body that distribute the flow of life force or *prana* from the surface to the inner recesses of the physiology. In Vedic martial arts, the task of a fighter was to attack or defend these gateways that hold the body's energy intact. To prepare for battle, preparatory exercises were designed to strengthen the connection between the vital points and the energetic core of the body. These exercises remain alive today in the South Indian *kalari* tradition of martial arts and in the *vinyasa* style of yoga.

Sushruta's work formed the basis of the medical system of Ayurveda, which developed alongside the Vedic martial arts tradition. Originally, Ayurveda was vibrational medicine and *vaidyas* (Ayurvedic physicians) routinely prescribed the chanting of Sanskrit *mantras* to prevent illness or treat specific ailments, regarded as energetic imbalances. In Ayurveda, the 107 vital points (*marmas*) of *Dhanurveda* are associated with specific Sanskrit syllables that enliven their energetic current and promote health. By intoning the pure sounds of Sanskrit and regulating the breath, the *marmas* absorb the healing vibrations, directing them to the inner core of the body via the channels of the subtle nervous system to restore balance.

Finally, through the lore of his students, I learned that the great grandmaster of modern yoga, Sri Krishnamacarya, instructed his disciples to chant the entire Sanskrit alphabet while holding themselves in yoga *asana*. This rigorous practice not only kindles the inner fire, but strengthens the channels of *prana* held in the proper alignment of *asana*.

In light of all my findings, especially in *Dhanurveda* and its survival in the South Indian martial arts and yoga practices (the region that Krishnamacarya hailed from), I discovered a profound reason to pronounce the Sanskrit names for the yoga postures: *To awaken and enliven the inner core of the body, leading to effortless meditation and the attainment of samadhi.*

Pronouncing the Sanskrit name for the posture and feeling its energetic flow, therefore, is the power behind your yoga practice to achieve its ultimate goal, *samadhi*. Despite my initial skepticism, I now appreciate the absolute necessity of pronouncing the Sanskrit names of the *asanas* themselves as a portal to the spiritual freedom that yoga promises.

---

*A complete description of the marma points, their matching Sanskrit syllables and the pronunciation of the most significant yoga postures is provided in my comprehensive program, **Feeling the Alphabet of the Body**™. It is advised, however, that you first master the necessary basics of Sanskrit pronunciation and cultivated awareness of the subtle body and its structures presented in my **Feeling the Shakti of Sanskrit**™ and **Sanskrit for Yogis**™ programs.*

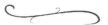

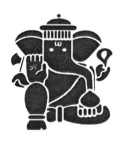

Chapter Three
Identity of Meaning and Feeling in Sanskrit

"Feel the Presence in the heart: not in the front, not in the back, not in the side, not above, and not below, but in the core of the very existence." ~ **Sri Sri Ravi Shankar**

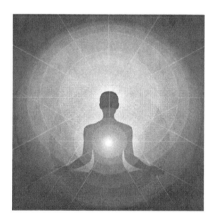

In a modern language like English, you have to add feeling or emphasis to the words you speak in order to express the meaning you desire to convey. For example, I can say, "I love you," with passion, with sarcasm, with tenderness, or with anger. The words themselves don't exhibit feeling. You have to add that yourself to articulate what you wish to communicate emotionally. You can also conceal what you really feel by manipulating the tone and emotion of your words.

In Sanskrit, however, meaning and feeling are identical. You can't pronounce a Sanskrit word perfectly without transmitting a specific feeling that arises from its syllables. Its vibrations, like music, present a feeling to the nervous system that cannot be altered or denied. That feeling naturally triggers a meaning.

Chanting and listening to the pure vibrations of Sanskrit awaken a profound inner feeling triggered by speaking and hearing. Higher states of consciousness increase through continuous and refined sensory contact. The Vedic teachings hold that by developing our most sensitive and subtle sense of hearing, our knowledge capacity expands.

In Vedic education, you don't learn a subject by making reference to sources outside yourself. Instead, knowledge results by awakening your own inherent capacity to know everything within your highly sophisticated nervous system. Neuroscience claims that we only utilize ten percent of our brain's capability. The feeling that a certain vibration generates within you simply helps to awaken the remaining ninety percent that's lying dormant. For example, if I want to understand algebra I simply need to enliven my capacity to know algebra that already exists within my intelligent nervous system.

For this reason, the sacred teachings of yoga are not "read" like books in English, but are "felt," arousing your own intrinsic faculty to know through the vibrations of Sanskrit. To culture "feeling intelligence," all the important scriptures were always composed in Sanskrit and orally transmitted from teacher to student. Each word in Sanskrit opens a new pathway of feeling, allowing a student to relate with whole body, mind and breath to the subject. All intelligence, therefore, is emotional intelligence.

INTRODUCTION TO THE SACRED LANGUAGE OF YOGA

What Western academics describe as Sanskrit "texts," like Patanjali's *Yoga Sutras*, therefore, are not the same as published books. We read books objectively, not experiencing the words with all of our senses beyond the sense of sight. When we read words on a page, our mind creates a division from the words themselves and what we interpret them to mean. In contrast, when you listen and repeat the Sanskrit words of a "text," your feeling capacity allows you to totally identify with the subject, expanding your range of perception and knowledge about it. For this reason, all the liberating knowledge throughout the history of India was always memorized orally.

It's said when Alexander the Great conquered northeastern India, he approached the most learned man he could find. "Bring me all your books," Alexander commanded, "for I wish to house them in my great library." The scholar obliged by presenting him with a basket full of decaying palm leaves. Alexander was very disappointed. "After all I have heard about India's great intellectual achievements, this stinking heap is all you have to show for them?"

The learned man listened patiently to Alexander's rants and then responded, "We need not contain our sacred knowledge in books. Everything is inscribed perfectly in our hearts by memory."

Always passed down orally from teacher to student, the *Yoga Sutras* in Sanskrit embody a state of consciousness with a distinct feeling that's communicated to your nervous system via the sound of the *sutras*. By listening to and repeating the ordered syllables that make up the first chapter of the *Yoga Sutras*, for example, you attain the state of yogic union or *samadhi*. You don't objectively contemplate the philosophical principles expressed in the text. Instead, the precise arrangement of the syllables unfolds the actual goal of yoga in your nervous system.

In contrast, when you read or listen to the *sutras* in English translation, the intended feeling is entirely lost. For example, the first *sutra* is often translated, "Now begins the discipline that is yoga." The only meaning that line conveys to us is that a subject is being introduced to preface a more meaningful discussion to come later. There is no feeling that arises in you from these words except perhaps boredom.

Yet in Sanskrit, the first word of any scripture embodies the precise meaning and feeling of what it expounds. In the *Yoga Sutras*, the goal of the first chapter is to establish the yogi in the heightened state of *samadhi*. The meaning and feeling of the first word, *atha*, communicates the experience of *samadhi* directly to the nervous system.

Take a moment to experience this principle.

The first syllable of *atha* is pronounced "uh." Say that sound a few times, contrasting it with "aah." When you say "uh," you feel a contraction inside. In contrast, "aah" creates a feeling of release and expansion. You don't say, "Uh, I'm in love." You say instead, "Aah, I'm in love," and, "Uh, I stubbed my toe!"

"Uh" is a contraction. Because it's a contracting feeling, it communicates the meaning "no," "not" or "negation." It's like in English when we say something is "atypical." It means it's "not typical."

"Uh" is the first vowel of the 16 vowels of Sanskrit, each one corresponding to the 16 phases of the waxing/waning moon. Each phase of the moon has a particular emotional quality associated with it that's communicated via a vowel sound in Sanskrit.

The first syllable of *atha* correlates with the new moon. During the new moon phase we experience an absence of light. With that absence, we can see the totality. We see the fullness of the sky and stars in the cosmos.

Likewise, when we contract deep inside ourselves with the sound, "uh," we're pulled beyond the limitations of this gross physical form. We experience a state of pure being and inner freedom. Even though it connotes something negative, "not, negation or no", it really has to do with "not this." You are not your body, your feelings, or your thoughts. Rather you're part of something much deeper and much more expansive on an inner level. That's "uh."

The next syllable of *atha* is "tha." It's not like "tha" in "thank you." In Sanskrit, you pronounce this sound by bringing the tongue in-between the teeth. Then you drop the jaw straight down like a ventriloquist doll, "thuh."

As you repeat this sound, the energy feels like it's being pulled down. When you drop something, the force of gravity causes it to fall. "Thuh" both feels and means "gravity," which is the cause for your bondage to the earth.

Together, if you say "uh-thuh" it feels and means "no gravity," "not bound" or "no bondage." It means and feels like freedom. If you aren't subject to the laws of gravity, you're liberated. When are you free? Are you free when you mind is stuck in the past? Or when you're projecting onto the future? You're free right now, in this moment. That's why the translation of *atha* is "now."

The goal of yoga is summarized and experienced in that first word. If you can feel the pulse of the present moment contained in the Sanskrit word *atha*, you're established in the state of union that is yoga. You're totally and perfectly free. The remaining *sutras* unfold the experience of the present moment so you can easily recognize it instinctively when your mind takes you out of the state. The *Yoga Sutras*, therefore, contain the vibrational code that allows you to attain *samadhi* effortlessly within your own body and mind through the vehicle of Sanskrit as sacred sound.

---

*To engage in the traditional transmission of yoga's most sacred "texts" in Sanskrit, I recommend my **Sanskrit & Yoga Mastery**™ program that instructs you in the rules and practice of Vedic chanting and awakens you to the true meaning and feeling inherent in the Upanisads, the , and the Bhagavad Gita. Preliminary mastery of the material in **Feeling the Shakti of Sanskrit**™ and **Sanskrit for Yogis**™ is required for enrollment.*

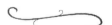

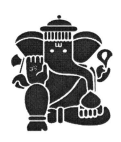

Chapter Four

Pronunciation of the Sanskrit Syllables and the Preservation of Prana

"When we think of a particular letter of the Sanskrit alphabet or a combination of these letters, each produces certain thoughts, certain mental vibrations...Each syllable has within it a particular ray of consciousness."
~ Swami Veda Bharati

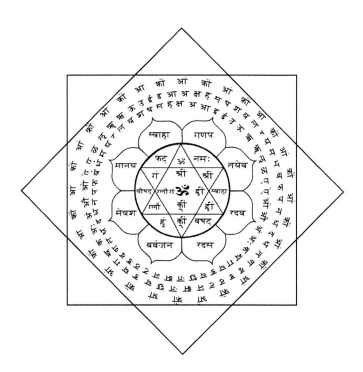

There's a noticeable difference between spending an hour speaking in English and an hour chanting in Sanskrit. In the former case, you find your energy depleted. That's because we have no mechanism in our modern languages to recapture the life force that gets expelled with our exhalation as we speak. In the latter case of Sanskrit, however, the simple rules of pronunciation are designed to redirect the *prana* back into the physical and subtle body.

As you exhale through your mouth, you'll notice that the breath passes over five distinct regions: the larynx, the soft palate, the hard palate, the teeth, and the lips. Each sound made in Sanskrit stimulates one of these regions, which are each a *marma* point. They open *pranic* pathways (*nadis*), that redirect energy that would otherwise be exhaled back into the subtle body. Speaking in Sanskrit, therefore, serves as a powerful form of *pranayama* that preserves and enlivens your life force.

Unlike most modern languages, the arrangement of the Sanskrit alphabet follows the evolutionary scheme of nature. While its vowels correspond with the "states" of higher consciousness and what some religions have described as the "angelic" realms, the consonants replicate the myriad of earth's life forms, from the amphibian, insect, bird, rodent, to the mammal kingdoms. Since humans are the only creatures who can recreate all the sounds of nature through our unique organs of speech, the voice serves as a bridge, connecting the body with the whole of nature, which is yoga. While our language often promotes misunderstanding and conflict, Sanskrit, when pronounced precisely, best achieves the ultimate goal of yoga practice — the total union of opposites.

Vowels form the core of Sanskrit's alphabet. These sounds are made without the assistance of the organs of speech (the tongue, the teeth, or the lips). Babies in their most innocent state of consciousness intone vowel sounds — "aaah," "eeeh," "oooh." At some point in our early childhood (around the "terrible two's"), we experience separation from our mother and say our first consonants — "maah" and "daah." (Or more often, "me!") The duality of consonants ("to sound together") expresses the psychology of our separation. As distinct individuals, we often find ourselves in life attempting to be understood, to connect with others and our world. This is why if we have a good conversation with someone, we say, "I connected with so-and-so." Or, if not, "We had a disconnect."

But the Sanskrit language recognizes that just as consonants are the sounds of separation, they also serve to re-connect us to the innocent state of unity we experienced as infants. For this reason, Sanskrit is called the "mother of all languages," because it returns us to the source of life, which according to the yogic point of view is silent, pure being.

This is how it works:

The Sanskrit vowels and consonants are found to be especially soothing to the mind and nervous system. They are most often "natural" sounds we make as we inhale and exhale, such as *so* (inhale) and *ham* (exhale). As the breath travels out of the body, we make language when the organs of our speech — the larynx, the base of the tongue, the tip of the tongue, the teeth, and lips — touch these five regions that connect mind with body. When precisely pronounced, the consonant sounds of Sanskrit penetrate these nerve centers in the head cavity like an acupuncture needle, directing *prana* to their corresponding body parts and nerve centers.

Mouth

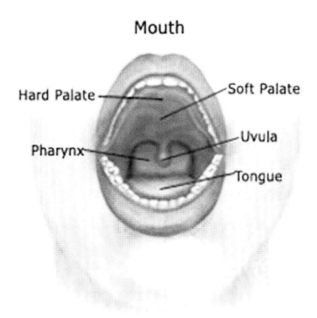

Hard Palate — Soft Palate

Pharynx — Uvula

Tongue

1. The *Guttural* region is in the throat.

2. The *Palatal* region is across the roof of the mouth or "soft palate."

3. The *Retroflex* region is located on the "ridge" or "hard palate" just before the teeth.

4. The *Dental* region is when the tip of the tongue makes contact with directly with the upper teeth.

5. The *Labial* region is through the lips.

Just as there are five regions and organs of speech, there are five energetic centers in the body, from the base of the spine to the throat. Each one of these centers resonates with the energies of the five elements (earth, water, fire, air, and ether), the five animal kingdoms (amphibian, insect, birds, rodents, and mammals), and the five classifications of Sanskrit consonants. By recreating the sounds of our world, we align ourselves with the rhythms and melodies of nature. We also do this when we practice yoga *asanas*, which also often mimic the animals of the natural world (cobra, frog, fish, eagle, elephant, and so on).

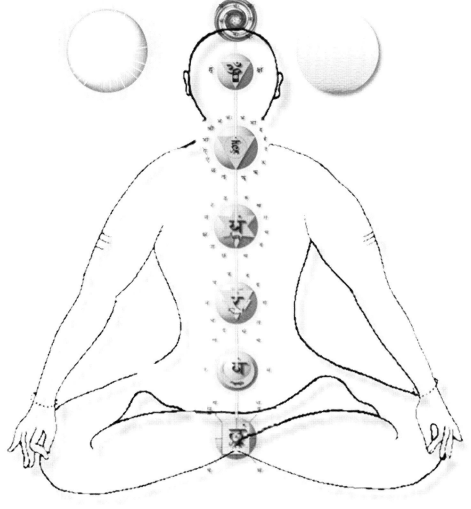

The Sanskrit Syllables and the Subtle Body Anatomy

Every Sanskrit syllable, therefore, opens the *marma* points in your vocal cavity and along the surface of your body, to direct *prana* through the channels or *nadis* that connect the *marmas* to the deep internal energetic centers or *cakras*. They also establish a resonance between the vibrations of your subtle body and the forms in nature that correspond with the Sanskrit syllables at their core.

As I mentioned earlier, the 16 vowel sounds link your emotional states with the phases of the moon. The 25 consonants connect your five sense organs with the five regions of speech, the five ways of sensing, the five sense objects, and the five elements in nature. The four semi-vowels orient you to the four directions in nature and link the flow of your spinal fluid with the upward flow of sap in trees and plants. The three sibilant sounds enliven the three nerve channels along the central axis of the body: the *ida, pingala* and *sushumna nadis* that intersect at the location of the seven *cakras*. The two final sounds allow your body, mind and breath to dissolve back into the primal state of unified consciousness at death.

The following page displays a simple chart of the arrangement of the Sanskrit syllables:

The Fifty (50) Sanskrit Letters of the Alphabet

- *14 Vowel Sounds + Anusvara and Visarga = 16*

अ	आ	इ	ई	उ	ऊ	ऋ	ॠ	ऌ	ॡ	ए	ऐ	ओ	औ	अं	अः
a	ā	i	ī	u	ū	ṛ	ṝ	ḷ	ḹ	e	ai	o	au	aṁ	aḥ

- *5 Classes of Consonant Sounds of Which There are 5 Varieties = Total of 25*

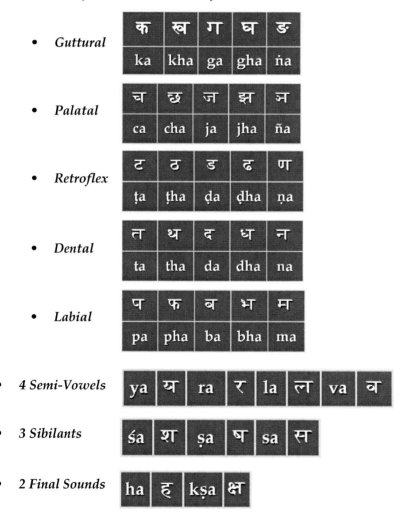

- **Guttural**

क	ख	ग	घ	ङ
ka	kha	ga	gha	ṅa

- **Palatal**

च	छ	ज	झ	ञ
ca	cha	ja	jha	ña

- **Retroflex**

ट	ठ	ड	ढ	ण
ṭa	ṭha	ḍa	ḍha	ṇa

- **Dental**

त	थ	द	ध	न
ta	tha	da	dha	na

- **Labial**

प	फ	ब	भ	म
pa	pha	ba	bha	ma

- *4 Semi-Vowels*

ya	य	ra	र	la	ल	va	व

- *3 Sibilants*

śa	श	ṣa	ष	sa	स

- *2 Final Sounds*

ha	ह	kṣa	क्ष

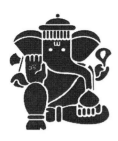

Chapter Five
Devanagari: The Sacred Calligraphy of Sanskrit

"Writing is divine, inherently holy, with powers to teach the highest mysteries; writing is the speech of the gods, the ideal form of beauty." ~ **John Stevens**, *Sacred Calligraphy of the East*

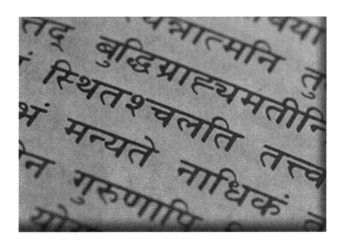

During one of the years I lived in India, I found myself traveling by open jeep through the interiors of Madhya Pradesh, which at the time was India's largest and least developed state. On pilgrimage to the source of the holy Narmada River at Amarkanthak, I had to traverse through many thick jungles, unpaved roads, and up steep inclines to get there…and through regions, my driver warned me, populated with man-eating tigers!

I didn't have the chance to encounter one of these magnificent beasts, but I met instead some really colorful characters along the way. In particular, one group of people who call themselves *Ram Namis* ("Those Rapt in the Name of God") made a deep impression on me.

These people express their devotion to their chosen expression of God, Lord Ram, by tattooing his name in the Sanskrit script, *devanagari*, all over their bodies. They print it on the fabric of the clothes they wear. The walls in their homes are covered with God's name. And they keep their mind solely focused on the Divine by continuously repeating, "Ram, Ram." In these ways, they saturate themselves with the presence of God -- from skin to soul.

This practice is in imitation of Lord Ram's best devotee, Hanuman, who when questioned if he really had any faith in God, tore open his chest to reveal the name of Ram permanently etched on his heart. Likewise these villagers believe that by tattooing their entire bodies with the letters of

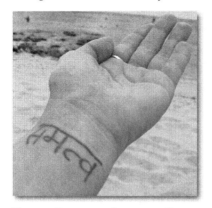

Photo Courtesy Susanne Draper,
Tatoo Design By Dr. Katy Poole

Ram's name, they become one with him. This is, in part, due to the geometric energy of the Sanskrit letters written in the *devanagari* script.

Devanagari, meaning "divine" (*deva*) and "city" (*nagari*), refers to one of the systems used to write down the oral Sanskrit syllables. Sanskrit can be written in any script (including the Roman script we use to read English) provided it accounts for all the nuances of its distinct sounds.

The word, *devanagari*, translates as "city of the gods," or more loosely, "the container of divine light." Because of its precision, beauty, and depth, the Vedic sages believed Sanskrit did not evolve out of ordinary human experience, but was the very speech of the gods or "beings of light" (*deva/devi*). It's the language with which the laws of nature and highly enlightened yogis communicate with each other and which describes the divine design of the cosmos itself.

The Sanskrit characters written in *devanagari* are, therefore, the outer symbols that express the intercommunication between human and divine. In

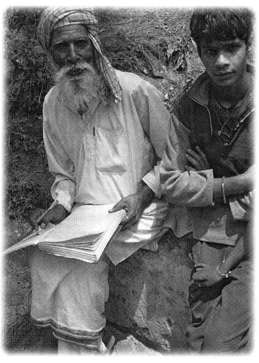

the ancient days, *devanagari* adorned temple walls to attract the gods to earth as well as to inspire humans toward their unified nature. This is why *devanagari* is also called "divine temple writing." It's a kind of sacred graffiti.

Writing the Sanskrit letters in *devanagari* is a sacred practice called *likhta japa* ("repetitive writing meditation"). The order of the strokes especially disciplines the mind to recognize specific flows of *prana*

Likhta Japa-Wallah, Garwahl, India

through the body and in nature. It trains you to recognize through eye/hand coordination the movement of energy currents pulsing through everything in creation.

The shapes of the script have a kind of musical quality to them, like Western musical notation, that conveys the movement of primordial sound. Although much of this knowledge is lost to us in the modern age, the shapes of the letters serve as pictographs for all the spiritual and terrestrial objects of the universe.

For example, *Om* as it is written in *devanagari* conveys the shape of Shiva Nataraja, the law of nature that dances this world into being, that activates the three movements of life (creation, maintenance and destruction), and that sustains the three aspects of matter (purity, activity, and inertia). For this reason, he is also called Omkareshvara, "The Lord Who Creates the *Om*."

Compare the *devanagari* symbol with the image of Shiva Nataraja and see if you can discover the remarkable similarity in the forms of each.

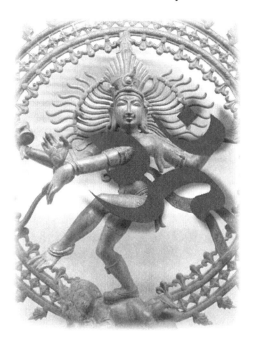

You can see that Shiva's limbs that extend to the left are like the three limbs of the first part of *Om:*

His open hand to the right holds either the fire or drum of creation and is indicated by the tail pointing to the right in the *Om* symbol:

ॐ

The crescent Moon that rests as a still point in Shiva's wild mane of hair is shown by the *candra bindu* (Moon drop) placed on top of *Om* pronounced as *anusvara* (nasalization)*:*

The circle of flames surrounding Shiva is the light of creation and the fire of destruction as in the first syllable of *Om*—**A**:

अ

Your own body is a vibrating mass of sonic shapes in the form of perfect geometry or *yantra*. *Yantras* consist of specific arrangements of geometrical shapes – circles, squares, and triangles -- that expand your consciousness visually in the same way *mantras* do aurally. *Yantra* is visual *mantra*, embodying the inner, vibratory nature of creation.

The *devanagari* characters are *yantras*. The human body is a *yantra*, an intricate matrix of nerves and paths of energy. Your breath follows a pattern that forms a perfect shape. It is said that the whole world is a *yantra* in which all the shapes of the mountains, flowers, rivers, and clouds tell us the story of creation. The *devanagari* letters, just like the Sanskrit oral syllables, provide a meditative glimpse into the sublime beauty of nature's arrangement.

Following is a sample of the Sanskrit vowels in *devanagari* with the order of their strokes indicated:

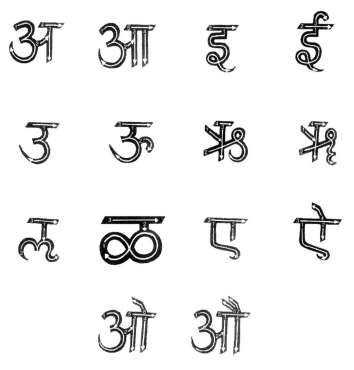

Sanskrit Vowels Written in Devanagari with Order of Strokes

For more detailed instruction on writing and reading all the Sanskrit characters in *devanagari*, I recommend you enroll in my comprehensive **Sanskrit for Yogis**™ program.

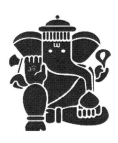

Chapter Six
The Bliss of Chanting Sanskrit as Mantra

*"As one continues to chant, the mind becomes saturated
with the mantras and easily achieves one-pointedness. The
heart is stabilized on its goal and begins to taste the joy
which is the inner essence of the mantras…One realizes that
the heart is the abode of deep peace, where love gushes."*
~ Swami Muktananda

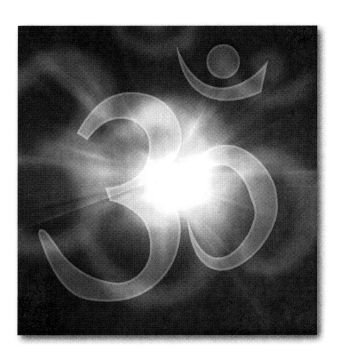

E very one of the 50 syllables in the Sanskrit alphabet is a *mantra*. Consisting of two parts -- "*man*" and "*tra*," -- *mantra* means, "that which extends (*tra*) the mind or heart (*man*)." *Mantra* establishes tranquility in mind and body by regulating the rhythm of the breath and silences the fluctuation of thoughts until only the feeling of the Sanskrit syllable exits. In this way, *mantra* is, as yoga scholar Georg Feuerstein describes, "a vehicle of transcendence."

Just as *mantra* establishes resonance with the created world, it also serves as a vehicle for the mind to come to rest. For the mind, according to the *Hatha Yoga Pradipika*, is "like a serpent, forgetting all its unsteadiness by hearing the mantra, it does not run away anywhere." Because the mind likes to "chew" on things, by repeating a *mantra* again and again, it becomes absorbed in it and forgets all other thoughts. The resulting peace is so tangible by its sheer contrast to the restless chatter of the mind, we remember it, especially during moments of duress when we find we can remain remarkably calm.

The repetition of *mantra* is called *japa*, which means "to whisper." There are three stages of *japa* that lead from the gross physical body to our innermost core of silence. First, the *mantra* is repeated out loud according to the rules of Sanskrit pronunciation. (The preferred number of repetitions is 108, the number required to purify all 72,000 nerves in the body.) Next, the *mantra* is repeated silently with just the lips moving and with a faint whisper. Then the *mantra* is pronounced mentally. Finally the *mantra* is simply felt as the mind totally dissolves and a deeper form of awareness dawns. This is the state of *samadhi* Patanjali describes in the *Yoga Sutras*.

The vibrations of the pure sounds purify the yogi's *panchakosha*, or the "five sheaths of the body." The voiced *mantra* purifies the *annamaya kosha*, the layer that is made up of the food we eat. It is also called the "gross physical," or our skin, bones, tissues, organs, and so on. The whispered repetition purifies the *pranamaya kosha*, or the breath that is our life force. And the mental act of *japa* works on the *manomaya kosha* or our "mental body." One of the common obstacles yogis have to achieving silence in meditation is the constant and mundane activity of our thinking mind. But with the mental recitation of *mantra*, our thoughts become absorbed in the feeling of the Sanskrit syllables, stilling the onslaught of mental noise.

When the chatter in our mind ceases, we become aware of a deeper level of intelligence within us, which is the *vijnanamaya kosha* or the subtle intellect. Then the light of pure discrimination dawns. Discrimination allows us to choose that which is most pleasant and uplifting to us. Because the mind finds peace to be the most charming state, it naturally is led to it through the silence following the practice of *mantra*. When we become full of silent peace the mind rests in a natural, content, and happy state, which is the *anandamaya kosha*, or the "bliss-filled body." This is true meditation, the highest form of yoga.

The *mantra, Om,* is the best example to experience how the syllables of Sanskrit function to unite body, mind, and breath with the natural cycles of life. The Vedic seers believed that the world begins, sustains, and ends with the three syllables that make up the one sound of *Om*--A, U, and M. The *Mandukya Upanishad*, an ancient yogic text of wisdom, declares that, "AUM stands for the supreme Reality. It is a symbol for what was, what is, and what shall be."

Of all *mantras, Om* is the most spiritually charged. It is called a "seed" *mantra* or *bija*, because just like the seed contains the potential for the whole tree, the seed syllable *Om* contains the potential for the whole creation, its maintenance, and its dissolution.

Om is not a symbol, meaning that it points to something outside itself. For example, if we see a nation's flag it is a symbol for the nation. It is not the nation itself. But *Om* itself embodies all the four aspects of creation, maintenance, dissolution, and silence within the sounds that make it up:

> A = Creation, the Navel, the Creator god (Brahma), and the
>   Waking State of Consciousness
>
> U = Maintenance, the Heart and Lungs, the Sustainer god
>   (Vishnu), and the Dreaming State of Consciousness
>
> M = Dissolution, The Third Eye, the Transformer god (Shiva),
>   and the Deep Sleep State of Consciousness

Sages (and now some scientists) believe *Om* to be the primordial sound that created the universe. Yogis find when you intone "AUM" in your own body you reconnect with the source of creation. Because of its power to generate and rejuvenate life, *Om* is called *pranava* ("life force itself"). But the energizing effects of *Om* are better experienced than described.

Now experience the precise way Om enlivens the energy in your body and connects you to the larger forces of natural law:

Take a deep breath in and exhale by slowly releasing the sound, "aaaaah." If your breath is not shallow, you may notice a sensation in the abdomen.

The sound resonates in the same part of the body that is responsible for the creation of another life in women, the womb, and the digestion, which continuously replenishes our bodies with the life-giving nutrients in food throughout our lifetime. In Sanskrit, the vowel sound, "a" corresponds with the function of creation and the waking state of consciousness.

Now take another deep breath in and exhale the sound, "uuuuuh." You may notice a sensation in the upper chest area. This is the location of the heart and lungs, the organs essential to the circulation of blood and nutrients as well as the breath throughout the body. Without the constant beating of the heart and the in-and-out flow of breath, we would soon find ourselves dead. Like these organs, the Sanskrit vowel, "u" resonates with the maintenance function of the body and the dreaming state of consciousness. Just as the blood and breath pervade the body, when we dream our thoughts pervade the environment. And neuroscience is now discovering the importance of the dream state to physical and psychological health.

With a last full breath, release the sound, "mmmm." Feel how it vibrates in the head cavity, directly behind the center of the forehead. This is a very powerful region of the subtle physiology described as the "third eye" or the eye of wisdom. The final sound of *Om* is the most significant sound in the Sanskrit alphabet. It instills the life force in the *mantra*.

Remember when you were a kid and Mom made something delicious to eat. You would close your eyes and exclaim, "mmmm, good." Also when we come to the end of something, we often feel satisfied. According to yoga philosophy, creation begins with thought (and sound) and ends in contented silence. It is held that the soul enters the body through the top of the head and exits through the same entrance. The uppermost region of the body is associated with dissolution and corresponds with the Sanskrit vowel "m" (also called *anusvara*, or "nasalization") and the state of deep sleep.

Now put all three sounds together. As you breathe out, pronounce "AUM." Feel each of the sounds resonating within the three distinct regions of the body. At the end of several repetitions, simply observe the sensations in the body. You may notice the mind is more silent. This "sound of silence" is said to be the source of creation and the "fourth" state of consciousness, which is peace.

The fourth state (*turiya*) is the still point of the turning world. It was there before you were born, is with you now as the silent witness to your changing life, and will be present after you're gone. This is *samadhi*, which Patanjali insists is the pre-requisite to yoga. You don't practice yoga, therefore, to *attain samadhi*. Rather, it helps you to uncover what is already your natural state of being. So as one of my clever *Sanskrit for Yogis*™ students once announced after chanting *Om*, "May the *fourth* be with you!"

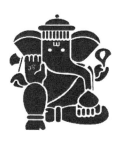

Chapter Seven
Technology of Sanskrit as Sacred Sound and Modern Science

"Knowledge of the supreme is spiritual wisdom and also science, including all its various branches. The earth, the sky, and outer space are the feet of that divinity whom humankind is trying to perceive with the eye of higher intelligence." ~ Swami Muktananda

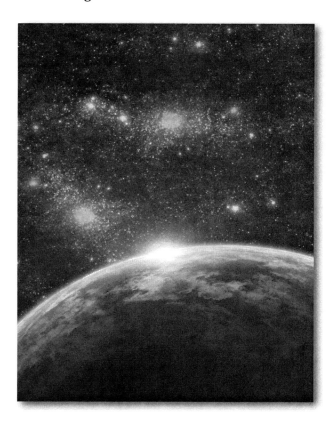

While yogis have known for centuries the healing and enlivening effects of *mantra* on body, mind, and spirit, scientists now corroborate this ancient auditory technology with modern research. The western medical community became aware of the effects of sound on the body with the discoveries made by Dr. Alfred Tomatis, the French medical doctor credited with first observing that fetuses respond to sound stimuli as they develop in the womb.

Serving as the physician for a Benedictine monastery outside of Paris, Dr. Tomatis was called to treat an outbreak of depression among the brothers. After questioning the monks, he learned that the new abbot had recently ended their daily ritual of Gregorian chanting. Dr. Tomatis concluded that without the auditory stimulation of the sacred chants, the monks' central nervous systems regressed into a depressive mode.

After reinstating the practice of group singing, their depression lifted. The results were so immediate that it led Dr. Tomatis to study other forms of sacred chants from world religions. His research culminated in the *Tomatis Method*, which he claims achieves higher measurements of intelligence through active listening.

Dr. Tomatis' work laid the foundation for the discoveries made by Dr. Susumu Ohno, the chief geneticist of the *Beckman Research Institute* in Duarte, California. Dr. Ohno ascribed musical notes to each of the six amino acids that make up the DNA. As he transcribed the arrangement of these notes by the DNA helixes in living matter, he observed that the sound patterns are not random, but actually consist of specific melodies. After hearing the melody of a particular type of cancer, Dr. Ohno theorized that its cure might be in realigning the body's melodies to literally a different tune.

And what about the effects of repetitive primordial sound on the brain? How does it impact our stress levels?

Our Reticular Activating System (RAS) that consists of a bundle of nerve fibers in the medulla oblongata (near the brain stem) is responsible for alerting the brain to the presence of new stimuli. They are the primitive responses we all have to protect us from the threat of danger. The RAS was very useful when we were hunters and gatherers, but in the post-industrial, high tech age we find ourselves bombarded by a continuous assault of noise and images that contribute only to the over-stimulation of our instinctual reactions. Instead of inducing heightened awareness, our brains become dull and unresponsive, inviting disease of both body and mind.

But when a stimulus, such as a *mantra*, becomes repetitive, the RAS grows accustom to it. Ted Melnechuk of the *Institute for Advancement of Health* claims that when a repetitive sound pattern is pronounced or played in the environment, the brain releases opiate-like endorphins as the RAS relaxes. Instead of inciting the brain to take immediate action, it calms it down instead.

And what about *Om*? Is there any scientific explanation that correlates with that offered by the yogis?

Dr. Ernst Rossi, M.D. suggests in his book, *The Psychobiology of Mind-Body Healing*, that language creates physiological changes in the body. The hypothalamus, located in the mid-lower level of the brain, "communicates" our language via the nerve fibers within the higher cortex to reach the various organs and systems of the body. In this way, the brain sends electrical patterns or brain waves throughout the entire bodily structure that correlate with specific mental and emotional states.

Just as there are three syllables that make up *Om*, brain waves are distinguished according to three types. Beta waves correspond with the waking state and are measured as heightened mental activity, such as we saw with the "*a*" sound of the *mantra*. The "dream state" of the syllable "*u*" mirrors the Alpha waves of the brain in a state of mild relaxation. And the "*m*" syllable that conveys complete satisfaction is experienced in the Theta state of deep relaxation that leads to meditative awareness or higher states of consciousness. Finally Delta brain waves (which scientists associate with dreamless sleep wherein ordinary awareness of "self" is absent) emit the pure silence of the *samadhi* described by the original yogis.

After teaching the yoga of sacred sound for many years, I've witnessed amazing incidences of healing that occurred after chanting Sanskrit, both physically and emotionally. Students shared that by opening the *pranic* pathways with Sanskrit, they found relief from headaches, insomnia, gastric distress, among other ailments. A student with MS symptoms practices reciting the alphabet daily to regain mobility. Emotional blocks also were released simply by liberating constrictions in the throat and other organs of speech which tend to hold emotional energy. Students suffering from debilitating depression found relief.

The experiences were so profound that one of my students, a pain management physician, plays recordings of Sanskrit *mantras* in his office for his patients. He reports that it has a positive impact on their stress levels. He even prescribes chanting *Om*!

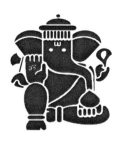

Conclusion
Sanskrit, The Next Step on Your Yoga Journey

"Chanting in Sanskrit is pure ambrosia, a sublime experience of precious vibration which gives profound inner peace. It is a song of praise to the divinity dwelling in the heart. It dispels illnesses and gives robust health, increases knowledge, strength, and fame, leading one to the realization of the Self of all."
~ Swami Brahmananda Sarasvati

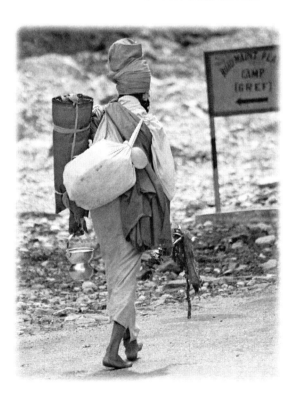

Now that you know the power of Sanskrit as a technology for awakening and expanding your consciousness, it's time to take the next step and experience it for yourself. For this aim, I've created a series of learning products to assist you in easily attaining the beautiful and transforming goal of yoga. These are not just classes where you learn some information. Rather they provide an opportunity for a profound experience to enliven your inner light.

For centuries, learning to chant Sanskrit and feel its primordial sounds have been at the basis of the Vedic, Yoga, and Tantra traditions. That's because of Sanskrit's power to tone and strengthen the subtle nervous system, making the body, mind and spirit fit for higher states of consciousness.

Yet there's a mistaken notion among yogis that Sanskrit is a dead, classical language that you think you probably should know something about but feel like it involves some kind of long and painful commitment to learn it.

That's what I thought over 20 years ago, which is why I enrolled in graduate school to study it in the academic way.

And truthfully?

I'd spend hours at a desk surrounded by thick books of grammar, pencil filings, erasure dust, and a pile of the hair I pulled out of my head trying to decode this incredibly intricate and complex language.

It wasn't until I sat with traditional Sanskrit teachers in Nepal and India that I realized there's a much more joyful and spiritually enlightened approach to derive the full-blown experience of Sanskrit as the actual vibration of your soul-filled consciousness — the same consciousness that allows you to read the words on this page as well as comprehend the intricate workings of the universe both seen and unseen.

This is why Sanskrit is the language of the *devas*, the universal principles of light that form the complete laws of nature. And it's the language of yoga because its 50 distinct sounds enliven and awaken your inner core — uniting body, breath, and spirit with the source of creation.

In the past, you had to be born into a family of Brahmin priests to experience this profound technology of higher consciousness, which is why few yogis in the West have access to Sanskrit as it is traditionally used in the practice of yoga and meditation in India. But now through the blessings of my revered teachers, you can derive the same benefits of sacred sound to bring more joy, light, and consciousness to your yoga and meditation practice.

To partake in the timeless transmission of Sanskrit, I recommend that you start with my introductory immersion, *Feeling the Shakti of Sanskrit*™, conveniently recorded to listen to anywhere at anytime. You'll learn the basic pronunciation of the Sanskrit syllables and experience their healing and enervating effects by imitating the sounds and vocal patterns without too much complicated explanation.

When you've gained sufficient comfort with the basics of pronunciation, you'll be ready to graduate on to the complete *Sanskrit for Yogis*™ home-study program. Through the teleconference classes, the detailed manual, workbook, and audio lessons, you'll gain both an exceptional foundational education in Sanskrit as it has been traditionally taught for centuries and a new approach to your yoga and meditation practice.

You'll experience how the precise pronunciation of Sanskrit cultivates the nervous system in preparation for profound meditation. You'll also discover Sanskrit's role in yoga's long tradition and why it's so important for yoga teachers and students to have access to this vital part of their practice. And finally, you'll be introduced to the ancient art of Vedic chanting and its contribution to all the sacred traditions of Yoga, Bhakti and Tantra.

With a solid foundation in *Sanskrit for Yogis™*, I invite you to participate in my more advanced programs. To assist yogis in not only pronouncing the Sanskrit names for the yoga postures, but also in experiencing their sonic shapes, you'll want to enroll in my *The Alphabet of the Body™* home study programs and teleconferences. And for a complete immersion into the art and science of Vedic chanting, the wisdom of the *Upanisads*, the enlightened technology of the *Yoga Sutras*, and the method and attainment of yoga's supreme goal of the *Bhagavad Gita*, I encourage your continued and deepened study in my *Sanskrit and Yoga Mastery Program™*.

My goal in creating state-of-the-art distance learning tools complemented with excellent instruction through webinar, teleconference, and live seminars is to give you life-changing exposure to the enlightening power of Sanskrit as it has always been taught throughout the centuries in India. Mostly, it's an opportunity to evolve your yoga practice from physical *asana* to a more rarified experience of transcendental light. I welcome you with all my heart to walk this sacred and transformative path.

Lokah Samastah Sukhino Bhavantu!
(May All Beings Be Happy!)

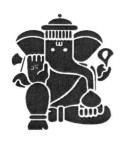

Acknowledgements

I must first of all acknowledge my husband, Sri Jeff Poole, for his tireless and devoted efforts to bringing Vedic knowledge out into the world. A dedicated teacher and practitioner of meditation for over 37 years, he first encouraged me to step down from the "ivory tower" of academia to share my knowledge of Sanskrit with the yoga community. My gratitude to him is oceanic and my love beyond galactic. None of what I do would even be remotely possible without his technical expertise, spiritual energy, and exquisite intelligence.

I am eternally grateful to my spiritual Guru, Sri Sri Ravi Shankar, who awakened my *jyoti* so that I could see far more than I ever imagined I could. I am grateful for the beautiful *ashrama*, Ved Vignan Mahavidyapeeth, he created in Bangalore as a safe haven for young Sanskrit students to preserve the traditional Vedic learning methods. I am grateful for all the years I spent in his presence and for giving me the courage and strength to stand on my feet and spread my light.

I owe a profound debt to Maharishi Mahesh Yogi and his brilliant articulation of the real value of Sanskrit in his *Apaurusheya Bhashya*, a commentary on the Vedas. Maharishi gifted the world by bridging physics and spirituality in his teachings on the Veda that he gained at the feet of his master, Gurudev Brahmananda Sarasvati. I am blessed to have touched Gurudev's holy sandals in May 2010 as they are housed at Jyotirmath in India. They remain inscribed on my heart as a living testament to the unbroken Vedic lineage of Adi Shankaracharya.

Special thanks to my academic teachers of Sanskrit – Mrs. Nandini Iyer and Gerald J. Larson – who no doubt may be in disagreement with some of the claims I make in this book, but to whom I am nonetheless indebted. I learned discipline and rigor from Professor Larson and that foundation has only served me in my life. To my traditional Sanskrit teachers I've already mentioned in the chapters of my book, I feel incredibly blessed by your generosity and faith in me. Thanks to the late Swami Lokeswarananda of the *Ramakrishna Mission* in Calcutta for granting me access to the Sanskrit resources and teachers at the *Institute of Culture* during the years I lived in that city. Thanks to my dear friend and research assistant, Dr. Babita Verma and her husband, Dr. Biswajit Mohanty, of Delhi University, for helping me to see the real heart of India. And I owe a special debt of gratitude to Pandit V. Shastryji who patiently and lovingly taught me the *Sri Suktam* one sultry Montreal summer and in doing so opened the door to the traditions of Tantra and Sri Vidya that I've just barely stepped through.

I extend special thanks to my family, especially my mother, Karin Komenda, who helped me tremendously earn my doctoral degree. I thank my sister, Julieane Frost, for first introducing me to the people and cultures of India by bringing exchange students home when she worked in the Education Abroad Program at Clark University. I feel blessed to have had the help and support of my sister, Christine Komenda, throughout my life in all my creative endeavors. And I'm grateful to my deceased father, John Komenda, for his childlike enthusiasm for all my adventures in Nepal and India. He loved hearing my stories when I'd return home and often stayed up into the wee hours of the morning asking me many questions about how Indian people eat, farm, and pray. If you're entertained by my storytelling, it's entirely due to my father who taught me well.

This book is a result of a simple course that I was asked to create for yoga teacher training by Heather Peterson of *Core Power Yoga* seven years ago. While the corporate officers of that yoga empire could not see the real value of Sanskrit, the thousands of students I taught in their many yoga teacher training programs certainly did. Their beautiful questions born from the beginner's mind brought out knowledge I never knew I had in me. They forced me to speak in language they could understand. They brought me down from my academic high horse and taught me to share simply and profoundly.

I am also inspired by my dedicated Sanskrit students – Francesca Jackson, Silke Schroeder, Jeanie Manchester, Selina Church, Becky Roskop, Amy Hansen, Lynne Minton, Shelley Cassidy, Candace Kirchner, Lori Pusateri, Jaimie Epstein, Randy Carlson, Katrina Gustafson, Lisa Schlelein, Shere Dayney, Sonja Picard, Shannon Dorato, Michelle Anderson, Shannon Earthtree, Jeri Steppat, Mindy Arbuckle, Eric Johnson, Smriti Ananda, Callae Gedrose, Kendall Wilson, Laura Riggs, Marley Vigdorth, Ellin Todd, Shaza Phillips, Judy Cannon, Yukiko Hunter, Jennifer Pierson, Pam Burgess, Clara Lazaroff, Brenda Campbell, Renay Oshop, and Louise Sanchez – who are truly the first drops in the "ocean of ladies" (and men!) I'm apparently destined to teach. There are many other students too numerous to mention who I also hold dear, but these students are truly the pioneers. It's easy to follow a trend, but much more courageous to forge one.

I must also acknowledge the Boulder/Denver area yoga centers and their directors where I was invited to teach *Awakening with Sanskrit*™ in their yoga teacher training programs over these past years: Katrina Gustafson of *Karma Yoga Center*, Jeanie Manchester of *Anjaneya Yoga Shala*, Annie Freedom of *Samadhi Center for Yoga*, Shannon Paige Schneider of *OmTime*, Michelle Anderson of *Studio Be*, Rebecca Baack of *Core Power Yoga*, and Heather Peterson and Dave Porter of *Core Power Yoga*.

I also wish to thank Carlos Pomeda for sharing my work with his students in Europe and Lynne Minton for inviting me to share Sanskrit with her yoga students in Alaska. Finally, without the support of great friends I'd be lost. Thanks especially to David Corell, Marise Cipriani, and Kabir Chalfin.

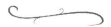

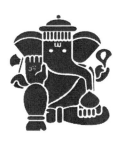

Glossary

"Like word and its meaning united,
For the right understanding of word and meaning,
I venerate the two parents of the universe,
Parvati and the supreme lord, Shiva." ~ **Kalidasa**

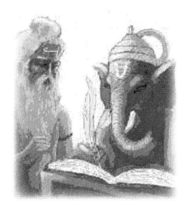

Abhinavagupta	Prolific *guru* of Kashmir Shaiva lineage (born 950 CE) famous for his composition of *Tantraloka* (12 volumes) and his deep insights on Sanskrit poetics, mysticism, philosophy, aesthetics, and phonematic emanation (theories on the expansion of sound).
Adi Shankara	Founder of Shankaracharya lineage of Advaita Vedanta (non-dualism); famed for his enlightened commentaries on the *Bhagavad Gita*, the *Brahma Sutras*, and also for his beautiful musical and poetic compositions such as *Shiva Manasa Puja, Saundarya Lahiri, Dakshinamurti Stotram*, among others.
anandamaya kosha	The bliss-filled sheath, covering, or layer of the subtle human body.
annamaya kosha	The sheath surrounding the body consisting of food; the flesh, blood, bones, etc.
asana	Presence, existence, one's silent abode, a quiet seat; anything that is done without interruption and with full attention, posture; the *Hatha Yoga Pradipika* lists 84 postures of the Yoga system, five of which are the most important: *padmasana, bhadrasana, vajrasana, virasana, svastikasana*.
bija	Seed, element, primary cause or principle; the source or origin of something; the true, underlying cause of anything coming into being.

bindu A detached particle or drop; the dot over a letter representing the *anusvara* (nasalization); sudden expression like a drop of oil in water expanding; the appearance of the universe from a sudden big bang; a tiny, concentrated drop of life; the center of any *yantra* (meditation diagram); the third eye center.

brahmana
(Brahmin) One who has divine knowledge; a priest; the name for a class of Vedic scriptures that contain rules for the use of *mantras* (where, when, by whom, and to which deity) and detailed explanations of their origins and meanings.

cakra Circle making, a potter's wheel, a circle or sphere, a cycle of years or seasons; the winding of a river, a whirlpool, an energetic sphere in the subtle body.

candra bindu A Moon drop, the archaic Vedic form of the *anusvara* that is contained within the *devanagari* syllable *Om* (ॐ).

deva Heavenly, shining; light-filled being; a deity, a god; a force responsible for a particular law of nature; one who sports or plays.

devanagari *Devanagari*, meaning "divine" (*deva*) and "city" (*nagari*), refers to one of the systems used to write down the oral Sanskrit syllables. The word, *devanagari*, translates as "city of the gods," or more loosely, "the container of divine light." The script most commonly used to depict Sanskrit characters, the outer symbols that express the intercommunication between human and divine.

devi	A female light-filled being; a goddess; an emissary of *shakti*; the feminine principle activating the creative processes of life.
guru	Heavy, weighty, difficult to digest, great, large, excessive, difficult, hard; a venerable and respected person, a teacher of the highest knowledge, a real "heavy dude."
manomaya kosha	The sheath or covering of the mechanical, thinking mind that surrounds the subtle body.
mantra	An instrument of thought, a potent prayer or string of Sanskrit syllables having the power to transform, enliven, and purify the body and environment; a sacred Sanskrit verse that makes up the sound form of a deity or law of nature; the inner or secret design of creation in the form of unfolding sound patterns.
marma	The Sanskrit word for *marma* means "mortal" or "vulnerable point" referring to tender, weak or sensitive access points located anatomically at sites where veins, arteries, tendons, bones or joints intersect. Localized vital energy points on the surface of the body that are infused with *prana* and imbued with consciousness, serving as acupoint bridges or doorways between the body, mind and soul. Affect the flow and balance of *prana* when stimulated to aid healing of vital organs.
nada	The sound of the vibration of the universe; the resounding echo of creation; the unfolding melody of existence.

nataraja	The lord of the dance, a name for Shiva who creates the world through the resonation of his thunderous *tandava* (foot stomps); the motion of his dance articulates the shape of a cosmic *Om* that activates the divine cycles of creation, maintenance, and destruction.
pandita *(Panditji)*	Learned, wise, skilled in something; a scholar, teacher or one who speaks about sacred things and subjects with divine authority.
prana	The breath of life, living spirit, total vitality within and without.
pranamaya kosha	One of the five sheaths or coverings surrounding the subtle body made up of vital life breath.
pranava	A name describing the *mantra Om*, meaning primordial sound that is the source of all life-force.
pranayama	The restraint or control of the life force (*prana*) in the body through the practice of measuring and conscious direction of the breath; the fourth limb of the eightfold yoga practice according to Patanjali.
rishi	A seer (and hearer) of the divine impulses of intelligence emanating from the source of creation; a singer of sacred hymns; a poet or sage; any person who alone or with others invokes the deities of nature using rhythmical Sanskrit speech; an awakened one who sees, hears, and repeats the Truth.
samadhi	Putting together, joining or combining, a union, a whole, an aggregate; completion, accomplishment, bringing into harmony; profound meditation; a kind of trance or suspension of ordinary consciousness; the eighth limb of the yoga path according to Patanjali; a sanctuary or tomb of a saint.

samskrita	Put together, constructed, well or completely formed; perfected, purified, consecrated, sanctified, hallowed, initiated, refined, adorned, ornamented, polished; the perfected language of pure consciousness.
shakti	Power, strength, might, ability, energy; the energy or active power of a deity personified as a divine feminine principle; the primal creative power; the great goddess who activates and causes the final dissolution of all life.
shiva	Auspicious, propitious, gracious, favorable; benign, kind, benevolent; the deity responsible for dissolution, destruction, transcendence and also creation.
shruti	That which was heard; a name for the Vedas that were divinely cognized by the ancient *rishis*; a stream, flow, or effusion of the melodious pure vibrations of consciousness that allow it to become manifest in creation.
sutra	Little thread, a sacred thread, a thread running through cloth holding it together; refers to the verses of a sacred work as in the *Yoga Sutras*, the smallest form of expression that only contains the most necessary words. They are called little threads based on the belief that it only takes a small thread of knowledge to save a person drowning in ignorance. Krishna said to Arjuna in the *Bhagavad Gita*, "*Even a small bit of this knowledge saves one from great fear and suffering.*"
upanisad	The sitting down at the feet of another to listen to her words; secret knowledge given in this manner, the mystery that underlies or rests underneath the external system of things, "secret doctrine"; a class of philosophical writings whose aim is the exposition of the secret meaning of the Vedas.

veda

Wisdom; true or sacred knowledge pertaining to the source, cause, and purpose of life; a collection of four divisions of knowledge: *Rig* (creation), *Yajur* (ritual maintenance of human life), *Sama* (celestial melodies of creation), *Atharva* (fire and Soma offerings to the ancestors); each of the Vedas has two distinct parts, *mantra* and *brahmana*. Together the *mantras* and *brahmanas* of the Vedas form the complete cognition of pure consciousness heard and seen by the *rishis*.

vijnanamaya kosha

One of five sheaths covering the subtle body made up of the intellect that regulates discrimination and wisdom.

yantra

An instrument either flat or three-dimensional composed of geometrical arrangements together with Sanskrit *mantras* used to induce meditation through the visual sense.

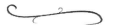

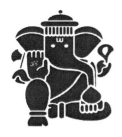

Index

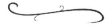

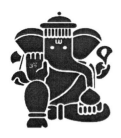

About Dr. Katy Poole

Yogini, Sanskrit scholar and Vedic Astrologer, Katy (Katyayani) Poole,

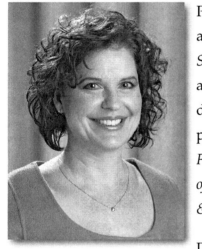

Ph.D. is the author of multiple books, courses and educational programs regarding *Sanskrit for Yoga*™ that are revolutionary and convenient home-study courses designed especially for Yoga & Meditation practitioners: *Awakening with Sanskrit*™, *Feeling the Shakti of Sanskrit*™, *The Alphabet of the Body*™, *Sanskrit for Yogis*™ and *Sanskrit & Yoga Mastery*™ *Program*.

Dr. Poole holds a doctorate in Religious Studies from the University of California, Santa Barbara and is founder of *Dr. Katy Poole: Vedic Astrology Life Insight* ™ *Coaching* (professional mentoring and coaching practice) and co-founder of *Shruti Institute for Vedic Arts (Shruti Inc.)* an educational institute dedicated to promoting, enlivening and preserving the ancient knowledge of Sanskrit (the Yoga of Sacred Sound), Jyotisha (Vedic Life Coaching), and Meditation (Vedic Mantras).

Websites: *http://www.ShrutiInc.com/*, *http://www.SanskritForYoga.com/*, *http://www.VedicAstrologyLifeInsight.com/*, *http://www.DrKatyPoole.com/*

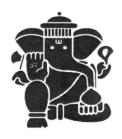

About Sanskrit For Yoga
Offerings: Books, Home-Study Courses, Programs and Live Events

Programs offered by Dr. Katy Poole:

Feeling the Shakti of Sanskrit™

The Alphabet of the Body™

Sanskrit for Yogis™

Sanskrit & Yoga Mastery Program™

For additional information send email or visit online locations:

Sanskrit For Yoga LLC:

- *info@SanskritForYoga.com*

- *www.SanskritForYoga.com*

Dr Katy Poole LLC:

- *info@DrKatyPoole.com*

- *www.DrKatyPoole.com*

- *www.VedicAstrologyLifeInsight.com*

S *anskrit for Yoga*™ aims to provide you with an excellent education in the most important and useful aspects of Sanskrit as they pertain to your growth and development as a yoga student or teacher. Using state-of-the-art systems and learning tools, *Sanskrit for Yoga* products will help you to:

- *Master Perfect Pronunciation, Tone and Feeling of Sanskrit*

- *Vitalize and Energize Your Body and Mind with Sacred Sound*

- *Increase Your Professional Skills and Knowledge as a Yoga Teacher*

- *Develop and Expand Your Yoga Practice with Chanting & Meditation*

Enliven Your Inner Core with Sanskrit

At the heart of yoga for 5,000 years, it's time you experience the power of Sanskrit. As you intone its 50 syllables, you'll enliven, awaken and strengthen your inner core, making your body, mind, and spirit fit for the higher stages of yoga.

Enrich Your Yoga Practice with Sanskrit

Move beyond the mistaken notion that Sanskrit is a dead, classical language requiring a long and painful commitment to learn. In a short time, you'll easily pronounce the names for the yoga postures, increase the depth of your breath, and cultivate new pathways for the flow of *prana* (life force) with the vibrations of Sanskrit.

Enlighten Mind, Body, & Spirit with Sanskrit

Yoga is not just a physical exercise. It achieves profound expansion of the mind and spirit through the technology of Sanskrit as sacred sound. The practice of Sanskrit recitation:

- Increases Mental Alertness

- Sensitizes Emotional Awareness

- Enables Effortless Silent Meditation

The Sanskrit for Yoga Difference

No other Sanskrit programs available today offer instruction in this essential component of your yoga practice and teaching as well as the programs of *Sanskrit for Yoga*™. Most currently available Sanskrit home-study programs burden you with academic rules of grammar and translation. These completely miss the true purpose and power of how Sanskrit functions and why it is so integral to yoga.

Sanskrit for Yoga™ programs directly immerse you in the practice of Sanskrit cherished by traditional yogis for thousands of years – as a technology for awakening and expanding your life force.

What We Provide:

Our primary objective with *Sanskrit for Yoga*™ is to enliven, enrich and enlighten yoga practitioners regarding the knowledge, essential value, and proper understanding of the technology of Sanskrit, the sacred language of yoga.

Sanskrit for Yoga employs modern online systems to deliver exceptional training programs providing instruction in the proper use and application of Sanskrit as a technology of consciousness. This enables us to deliver these profoundly effective programs direct to you, anywhere you are, at any time you choose to enjoy your study.

No other Sanskrit programs offer instruction in these essential components at the foundations of yoga practice and teaching, as our *Sanskrit for Yoga* programs provide. Our programs immerse you in the practice of Sanskrit in an intimate fashion that's been cherished by traditional yogis for thousands of years — as a technology for awakening and expanding your consciousness and *prana* (or life force). The practice of Sanskrit recitation increases mental alertness, sensitizes emotional awareness, improves listening, and enables effortless silent meditation.

Sanskrit For Yoga™ **Offers the Following Programs:**

Awakening with Sanskrit™ – *Introduction to the Sacred Language of Yoga.* Our introductory mini-course will help you to gain a foundation for understanding the role of Sanskrit as a technology of sacred sound and its power to energize and awaken your vital life force.

Feeling the Shakti of Sanskrit™ – *Experiencing the enlivening and enlightening effect of Sanskrit as the Language of Yoga.* Our first level Sanskrit course teaches you to pronounce and recite the Sanskrit alphabet to increase mental alertness, sensitize emotional awareness and enable effortless silent meditation.

Sanskrit for Yogis™: *Introduction to Nada – The Yoga of Sacred Sound.* Our in-depth and comprehensive home-study program builds on the foundation of Sanskrit gained from *Feeling the Shakti of Sanskrit*™

course. You'll gain additional instruction in the rules of correct pronunciation and the connection between the Sanskrit syllables, forms in nature, and its vibrational affects on the architecture of your subtle body. You'll experience how pronouncing the syllables awakens and strengthens your inner core, making your body, mind and spirit fit for the higher stages of yoga. You'll learn to read and write the *devanagari* script of Sanskrit. And, finally you'll be introduced to the art and science of Vedic chanting in Sanskrit as a powerful technology for meditation.

The Alphabet of the Body™ – A Comprehensive Guide to Learning the Sanskrit Names of the Yoga Postures. This is a course in learning the Sanskrit names for the yoga postures and provides instruction in sacred sound and the subtle body. The course instructs you in relating the anatomy of the subtle body (the *marmas*, *nadis* and *cakras*) to the 50 sounds of Sanskrit. You'll also discover how the names of the yoga postures in Sanskrit serve to establish an energetic flow of *prana* between the physical and subtle physical bodies. You'll not only master proper pronunciation of the yoga postures, but also deepen your experience of the subtle power of yoga.

Sanskrit & Yoga Mastery™ Program – A Comprehensive Advanced Sanskrit Program. Our program combines the best aspects of Dr Poole's academic training with her deep connection to the Vedic lineage and years and years of yoga and meditation practice to provide you with an opportunity to advance your yoga practice and teaching. Topics included in the series are:

Sanskrit Vedic Chanting — Enliven Your Spirit with Sacred Sound. Receive instruction in Vedic chanting using the six main rules of Sanskrit Vedic chanting as applied to several traditional sacred Vedic chants.

The Practice of Samadhi — an Experiential approach to Patanjali's Yoga Sutras: Padas 1 & 2. Receive the opportunity to both feel and experience the transformative effects of each of the **Yoga Sutras** in **Padas 1 & 2.** You'll gain access to the living and vibratory quality of Patanjali's *sutras* by chanting them in their original Sanskrit.

The Yoga of Bhagavad Gita™ — Discovering Your Svadharma (Highest Life's Purpose) Through the 3 Yogas of the Bhagavad Gita: Raja, Karma, & Bhakti. Explore the philosophical teachings that make up the core of yoga's tradition and practice to life by exploring the enlightening dialogue between Krishna and Arjuna and how it relates to your own experience and development as a yogi.

The Yoga of the Upanishads™ — Embodying and Incorporating Upanishadic Wisdom in Your Life and Practice. Provides the solid foundation necessary to derive the greatest advantage from your study of yogic knowledge, as well as to begin to integrate Sanskrit into your yoga practice and teaching.

The Yoga of the Vedas™ — Immersion in the Sacred Foundation of Yoga and All the Great Traditions of Self-Realization. Gives you an in-depth immersion in the enlightening content of the 4 Vedas (*Rig, Sama, Yajur* and *Atharva*) as well as the important Vedangas (limbs of the Veda) such as Jyotisha (astronomy and astrology), Vastu, and Ayurveda (health and wholeness).

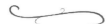

CPSIA information can be obtained at www.ICGtesting.com
Printed in the USA
LVOW131228240912

300042LV00001B/108/P